# SURGICAL ADHESIVES and SEALANTS

**HOW TO ORDER THIS BOOK**

BY PHONE: 800-233-9936 or 717-291-5609, 8AM–5PM Eastern Time

BY FAX: 717-295-4538

BY MAIL: Order Department
Technomic Publishing Company, Inc.
851 New Holland Avenue, Box 3535
Lancaster, PA 17604, U.S.A.

BY CREDIT CARD: American Express, VISA, MasterCard

BY WWW SITE: http://www.techpub.com

# SURGICAL ADHESIVES and SEALANTS

## *Current Technology and Applications*

**Edited by**

**David H. Sierra, MS**

Vice-President, Research and Development
Cohesion Corporation
Palo Alto, California

**Renato Saltz, MD, FICS, FACS**

Associate Professor of Surgery
Division of Plastic and Reconstructive Surgery
University of Utah
Salt Lake City, Utah

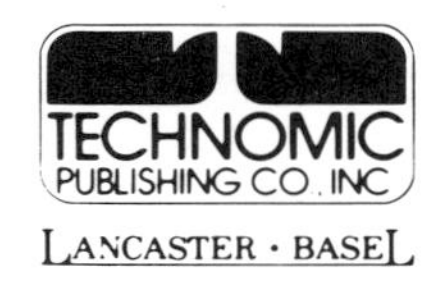


LANCASTER · BASEL

**Surgical Adhesives and Sealants**
a **TECHNOMIC** ®publication

*Published in the Western Hemisphere by*
Technomic Publishing Company, Inc.
851 New Holland Avenue, Box 3535
Lancaster, Pennsylvania 17604 U.S.A.

*Distributed in the Rest of the World by*
Technomic Publishing AG
Missionsstrasse 44
CH-4055 Basel, Switzerland



Printed in the United States of America
10 9 8 7 6 5 4 3

Main entry under title:
Surgical Adhesives and Sealants: Current Technology and Applications

A Technomic Publishing Company book
Bibliography: p.
Includes index p. 245

Library of Congress Catalog Card No. 95-61620
ISBN No. 1-56676-327-4

*This work is affectionately dedicated to my wife Karla*
*for her untiring support.*
*D. S.*

*To my wife Marcia, my parents Jayme and Berta*
*and my children Bianca and Felipe.*
*R. S.*

# CONTENTS

# PREFACE

Surgical tissue adhesives are an ancient idea, going back to the beginnings of recorded history. The concept of adhering, rather than suturing, packing, or stapling planes of tissue is attractive, in that it is fast-acting and assures complete closure. Numerous technologies have been tried; some with limited success, others outright failures. In short, the perfect adhesive does not exist. Limitations occur in a number of areas: strength, toxicity, degradation, and safety. It is also important to keep in mind that "one size fits all" does not apply to adhesives in surgical applications any more than it does in day-to-day application. As one would not use paper glue to seal a bathtub, one would presumably not apply an adhesive onto tendons, which is suitable for sealing corneas. The properties required of an adhesive for each indication are quite different.

Over the last twenty-five years, advances have been made in a wide range of technologies targeting some embodiment of a practical and safe adhesive. Foremost and most successful among these are cyanoacrylates, marine adhesive proteins, and fibrin-based sealants. Another promising adhesive technology is laser solders, a mixture of polypeptides and proteoglycans, which integrates with the repair site when laser energy is applied.

In light of these advances in the field, the *Symposium for Surgical Tissue Adhesives* was organized and held at the Atlanta Hyatt from October 8 – 10, 1993. The goal was to bring together these far-flung technologies in a comprehensive and cohesive manner. Presentations by investigators from around the world described the history of adhesives in medicine, current technologies, laboratory characterizations, and application developments, as well as regulatory aspects and clinical applications. We felt that as many viewpoints as possible, however conflicting, were important to present in order to give the most complete picture of the state of the art of surgical adhesives.

We owe a debt of gratitude to Katrinka Akeson, Dr. Gerald Chambers, and the staff of the Division of Continuing Medical Education at the Medical College of Georgia for their untiring support in putting together the symposium with us. Many thanks to Donna Scott, Erica Doster, PA-C, and Ingrid Heggoy for helping us to organize the symposium and the Division of Plastic and Reconstructive Surgery of the Medical College of Georgia for their support of this project. We also thank Dr. Luis O. Vasconez for his support, which allowed us to develop the earlier phases of the symposium, at the Division of Plastic and Reconstructive Surgery at the University of Alabama. We are grateful to the Plastic Surgery Educational Foundation for their endorsement to the symposium and to the generous financial contributions from our corporate sponsors and exhibitors. Finally, many thanks to the presenters at the symposium for their participation and contributions, especially those who authored the chapters in this book. We felt it was a fruitful and worthwhile effort. It is our sincere hope that the symposium participants and the reader will agree.

## CONTRIBUTING AUTHORS

N. Akhyani, *Plasma Derivatives Laboratory, American Red Cross, Rockville, Maryland*

P. Appourchaux, *Centre Regional de Transfusion Sanguine de Lille, Lille, France*

D. Arikan, *Maxillofacial Laboratory, Medical Center, Department of Veteran Affairs, Wilmington, Delaware*

I. Arikan, *Maxillofacial Laboratory, Medical Center, Department of Veteran Affairs, Wilmington, Delaware*

Lawrence S. Bass, *Institute of Reconstructive Plastic Surgery, New York University Medical Center, New York, New York*

A. Best, *Plasma Derivatives Laboratory, American Red Cross, Rockville, Maryland*

R. Brady, Jr., *Plasma Derivatives Laboratory, American Red Cross, Rockville, Maryland*

Theresa Brodniewicz, *Haemacure Biotech, Inc., Pointe-Claire (Montreal), Quebec, Canada*

T. Bui-Khac, *Haemacure Biotech, Inc., Pointe-Claire (Montreal), Quebec, Canada*

Thierry Burnouf, *Centre Regional de Transfusion Sanguine de Lille, Lille, France*

Miryana Burnouf-Radosevich, *Centre Regional de Transfusion Sanguine de Lille, Lille, France*

J. Camac, *Maxillofacial Laboratory, Medical Center, Department of Veteran Affairs, Wilmington, Delaware*

A. Campagna, *Plasma Derivatives Laboratory, American Red Cross, Rockville, Maryland*

William Drohan, *Plasma Derivatives Laboratory, American Red Cross, Rockville, Maryland*

P. Duval, *Centre Regional de Transfusion Sanguine de Lille, Lille, France*

P. Emire, *Haemacure Biotech, Inc., Pointe-Claire (Montreal), Quebec, Canada*

Dale Feldman, *Department of Biomedical Engineering, University of Alabama at Birmingham, Birmingham, Alabama*

B. Flan, *Centre Regional de Transfusion Sanguine de Lille, Lille, France*

William A. Fricke, *Center for Biologics Evaluation and Research, United States Food and Drug Administration, Rockville, Maryland*

Keith Green, *Department of Ophthalmology, Medical College of Georgia, Augusta, Georgia*

G. Grummon, *Plasma Derivatives Laboratory, American Red Cross, Rockville, Maryland*

S. Harding, *Plasma Derivatives Laboratory, American Red Cross, Rockville, Maryland*

R. Hennings, *Plasma Derivatives Laboratory, American Red Cross, Rockville, Maryland*

Harvey N. Himel, *Department of Plastic Reconstructive Surgery, University of Virginia Health Sciences Center, Charlottesville, Virginia*

J. Hollinger, *Plasma Derivatives Laboratory, American Red Cross, Rockville, Maryland*

J. J. Huart, *Centre Regional de Transfusion Sanguine de Lille, Lille, France*

C. Hue, *Plasma Derivatives Laboratory, American Red Cross, Rockville, Maryland*

Mark L. Kayton, *Department of Surgery, Columbia-Presbyterian Medical Center, New York, New York*

R. Kidd, *Plasma Derivatives Laboratory, American Red Cross, Rockville, Maryland*

C. Lasa, Jr., *Plasma Derivatives Laboratory, American Red Cross, Rockville, Maryland*

G. M. Lemole, *Maxillofacial Laboratory, Medical Center, Department of Veteran Affairs, Wilmington, Delaware*

G. Liau, *Plasma Derivatives Laboratory, American Red Cross, Rockville, Maryland*

Steven K. Libutti, *Department of Surgery, Columbia-Presbyterian Medical Center, New York, New York*

John F. Lontz, *Maxillofacial Laboratory, Medical Center, Department of Veteran Affairs, Wilmington, Delaware*

Martin J. MacPhee, *Plasma Derivatives Laboratory, American Red Cross, Rockville, Maryland*
Daniel Marchac, *Paris, France*
Gerald Marx, *New York Blood Center, New York, New York*
C. Michalski, *Centre Regional de Transfusion Sanguine de Lille, Lille, France*
Margaret Nowatarski, *Haemacure Biotech, Inc., Pointe-Claire (Montreal), Quebec, Canada*
Roman Nowygrod, *Department of Surgery, Columbia-Presbyterian Medical Center, New York, New York*
Hernan A. Nunez, *Plasma Derivatives Laboratory, American Red Cross, Rockville, Maryland*
Rodney C. Perkins, *California Ear Institute at Stanford, Palo Alto, California*
Janet B. Rodgers, *Division of Plastic Surgery, University of Kentucky, Lexington, Kentucky*
Kiti Rudnicka, *Haemacure Biotech, Inc., Pointe-Claire (Montreal), Quebec, Canada*
Renato Saltz, *Division of Plastic Reconstructive Surgery, University of Utah, Salt Lake City, Utah*
G. Savidge, *The Haemophilia Centre, St. Thomas' Hospital, London, United Kingdom*
Karl H. Siedentop, *Department of Otolaryngology—Head and Neck Surgery, University of Illinois at Chicago, Chicago, Illinois*
David H. Sierra, *Cohesion Corp., Palo Alto, California*
M. P. Singh, *Plasma Derivatives Laboratory, American Red Cross, Rockville, Maryland*
William D. Spotnitz, *Department of Thoracic and Cardiovascular Surgery, University of Virginia Health Sciences Center, Charlottesville, Virginia*
Julia K. Terzis, *Microsurgical Research Center, Eastern Virginia Medical School, Norfolk, Virginia*
Dean Toriumi, *Department of Facial Plastic Surgery, University of Illinois at Chicago, Chicago, Illinois*
Michael R. Treat, *Department of Surgery, Columbia-Presbyterian Medical Center, New York, New York*
Henry C. Vasconez, *Division of Plastic Surgery, University of Kentucky, Lexington, Kentucky*
J. M. Verderamo, *Maxillofacial Laboratory, Medical Center, Department of Veteran Affairs, Wilmington, Delaware*

## Symposium Corporate Contributors

American Red Cross
Rockville, MD

Centre Regional de Transfusion
Sanguine de Lille
Lille, France

Electromedics, Inc.
Englewood, CO

Haemacure Biotech, Inc.
Pointe-Claire, Canada

Miles Pharmaceutical Division
Berkeley, CA

Otogen Corp.
Palo Alto, CA

Stryker Blood Technologies
Kalamazoo, MI

ZymoGenetics
Seattle, WA

# SECTION I

# ADHESIVE TECHNOLOGIES

# *Chapter 1: History of Tissue Adhesives*

W. D. SPOTNITZ

## INTRODUCTION

It is beyond the scope of this work to detail comprehensively the history of tissue adhesives. However, it is valuable and appropriate to begin by reviewing the capabilities desired in an ideal adhesive. Then the abilities of the various available agents to attain these desired qualities will be assessed. The search for the perfect surgical "glue" is not complete, but as every surgeon knows, the applications for effective agents would be numerous. A broad spectrum of challenges, ranging from simple wound closure to control of massive hemorrhage awaits the competent adhesive. Such an agent would improve patient care, reduce morbidity and mortality, and potentially reduce health care costs.

## THE IDEAL ADHESIVE

The ideal tissue adhesive would have at a minimum the following capabilities. First, it would be *safe and biodegradable* so that no risks would be incurred by its use or the presence of its metabolites. Second, the agent needs to be *effective*. Effectiveness in tissue adhesives depends on tissue adherence strength, internal sealant bonding strength, hemostatic potential, tissue healing and regeneration characteristics, and infection control capability. Third, the material needs to be easily *usable*. Thus, the agent would need to be easily prepared and applied, initially malleable, and yet rapidly forming. Fourth, the adhesive needs to be *affordable* so that widespread clinical application would be reasonable. Fifth and finally, the agent must be *approvable* by government regulatory agencies for use in the United States. The modern tissue adhesives to be considered in this limited review include cyanoacrylate, fibrin sealants, gelatin-resorcinol-formol glue, mussel adhesive protein, prolamine gel, and transforming growth factor beta.

## CYANOACRYLATE

Initial work on these agents began in 1949 with Ardis [1]. Coover et al. characterized the adhesive properties of cyanoacrylate in 1959 [2]. The cyanoacrylates were used clinically in 1965 by Watson and Maguda for tympanic membrane repair [3]. The activity of these agents is based on their polymerization in the presence of hydroxyl ions [4] with the production of a solid adhesive and heat [5]. The glue is metabolized by hydrolysis to formaldehyde and alkylcyanoacetate that can be further metabolized and excreted in urine and feces [6]. Development of cyanoacrylate (Histoacryl®) and methyl-methacrylate (MMA) was investigated in an attempt to reduce tissue toxicity. The cytotoxicity of cyanoacrylate [5,7,8] is proportional to the dose used, and an association with liver sarcoma in animals has been reported [9]. Foreign body reactions, inflammatory and allergic responses, particularly dermatologic, can occur, and there is a question of carcinogenic potential.

Cyanoacrylates are strong adhesives capable of instantaneous bonding and rapid hemostasis. They can be easily applied as a single component glue system stored in a tube [6]. These adhesives have been used successfully in a wide variety of applications [10 – 17] including brain arteriovenous malformation embolization [18], retinal repair [19,20], and bone stabilization and sterilization [21].

Cyanoacrylate can be affordably priced and produced in reusable containers for convenience [6]. Further efforts are presently underway to reduce toxicity associated with the use of these agents [8]. The Food and Drug Administration (FDA) has not approved these compounds for widespread use as a surgical adhesive [6]. However, *n*-butyl-cyanoacrylate (Nexacryl®) is in the late stages of trials for the FDA approval in the treatment of scleral and corneal perforations. There have been individual case reports of complications with its clinical use [22,23].

## FIBRIN SEALANT

Fibrin was first used as a hemostatic agent by Bergel in 1909 [24]. Young and Medawar [25] initiated the use of fibrinogen as an adhesive in 1940 and Cronkite et al. [26] were the first to use the fibrinogen in plasma in combination with bovine fibrinogen as a biologic glue in 1944. Matras [27] increased the effective use of fibrin sealant in 1982 by using a concentrated preparation of fibrinogen.

Fibrin adhesive is manufactured from blood [28] and is thus associated with the risks of viral blood-borne-disease transmission. These dangers can be eliminated by using autologous sources of fibrinogen [28–34]. Commercial efforts at improving the safety of large pools of human plasma as fibrinogen sources have dealt extensively with a variety of viral sterilization techniques [35,36]. Fibrin sealant is an attractive surgical adhesive theoretically because it consists of biologic components of the natural clotting system [37]. Thus, it is biodegradable through routine fibrinolysis [38] and less likely to have any malignant potential.

In addition to the risks of viral transmission, fibrin sealant without accompanying antibiotics can serve as a bacterial growth medium potentiating infection. Recent reports suggest that bovine thrombin required for use with fibrinogen to produce adhesive can induce antibodies to thrombin and Factor V creating significant clotting abnormalities [39,40]. Bovine thrombin inoculation into the systemic circulation may have been the cause of hypotension and/or anaphylaxis seen with fibrin sealant use [41,42]. Human thrombin may soon be available to reduce the immunologic risks associated with bovine thrombin.

Fibrin sealant is formed when fibrinogen and thrombin are combined in the presence of Factor XIII and calcium as catalysts [38]. Other factors affecting the formation of this adhesive include pH, fibronectin, and temperature. Fibrin sealant is susceptible to fibrinolysis by endogenous or exogenous plasmin. Antifibrinolytic agents such as aprotinin can reduce the rate of fibrinolytic degradation of fibrin sealant [43].

Fibrin sealant is an effective hemostatic and adhesive agent. Its characteristics—specifically strength and rate of formation—are greatly affected by the concentration of fibrinogen and thrombin, respectively, employed [44]. However, the adhesive and critical glue bonding strength of this agent are limited when compared to synthetic chemical adhesive.

Because fibrin matrices are critical for effective wound healing, fibrin sealant acts to improve wound repair by serving as a scaffolding for fibroblast migration [38]. Fibrin sealant as it is fibrinolysed can serve as a carrier for the slow release of antibiotics or other agents which may be valuable in the wound-healing environment [45–47] or as chemotherapy for malignancies [48]. Fibrin sealant application has been used successfully in a large number of surgical specialties ranging from thoracic-cardiovascular [49] and neurologic [50] to head and neck [51] and ophthalmologic surgery [52]. The number of uses is extensive and ranges from hemostasis of vascular anastomoses [49] to securing split thickness skin grafts [53].

As a two-component adhesive, fibrin-sealant activity is based on thorough mixing of fibrinogen and thrombin [54]. The rate of glue formation depends on thrombin concentration. Thus, there is a learning curve in developing effective methods of applying fibrin sealant as well as choosing the specific rate of reaction desired for each use. In general, the agent is easily employed and is an effective tissue glue with a high affinity for collagen. However, there are limits to its adhesive strength.

Although they are not reusable [6], commercial forms of fibrin sealant are similar in price to cyanoacrylate. In addition, larger volumes of fibrin sealant may be required for certain larger surface area applications [49]. This may result in increased costs.

Although the overall clinical attractiveness of fibrin sealant is large, this agent has not been approved for use by the FDA in spite of many application attempts. The present regulatory environment seems to be an obstacle for approval of an agent that has even a remote possibility of blood-borne disease transmission. This has created a large demand in the United States for blood-bank fibrinogen production from either single-donor or autologous sources. This ''noncommercial'' fibrinogen is then used with bovine thrombin to create fibrin sealant.

## GELATIN-RESORCINOL-FORMOL (GRF) GLUE

This adhesive was developed and tested by Braunwald and Tatooles beginning in 1964 [55]. Guilmet achieved significant clinical application in the treatment of aortic dissections in 1977 [56]. GRF adhesive was initially reported to be free of significant associated risks, but recent reports suggest a danger of vascular tissue disruption [57].

The adhesive is formed from gelatin, resorcinol, and distilled water in the presence of formaldehyde, glutaraldehyde, and heat (45°C) [55]. This reaction produces a material that is particularly effective as a tissue adhesive. By eliminating abnormal tissue planes, this agent improves hemostasis but has no inherent capacity to promote wound healing. The ingredients of this adhesive need to be thoroughly mixed for thirty to forty-five seconds, resulting in the formation of a polymer that is the final adhesive material [58]. The field of application needs to be as dry as possible for successful use [58]. The most effective clinical applications of this agent have been in cardiovascular surgery where it has been used successfully in aortic dissection repairs [55,56,58]. The glue can be used to eliminate the dissection plane by gluing the layers of the aorta together and strengthening its wall to hold sutures more effectively. Gelatin-resorcinol-formol adhesive has also been used successfully to achieve hemostasis during hepatectomy and nephrectomy [59]. While the costs of this product are not prohibitive, it is not FDA-approved for commercial production.

## MUSSEL ADHESIVE PROTEIN PROLAMINE GEL AND TRANSFORMING GROWTH FACTOR BETA (TGF-$\beta$)

Because these three agents are in the early stages of development, they will be considered as one group.

Mussel adhesive protein is derived from the collagenous material produced by the mussel that allows the sea mussel (*Mytilus edulis*) to adhere to underwater surfaces [60]. It is a protein composed of seventeen amino acids containing unusual amounts of dihydroxyphenylalanine [61]. Although this adhesive is biodegradable, it is reported to have caused inflammatory responses upon intraocular injection [62]. The methods of purification and the characteristics of this biologic adhesive, as well as possible clinical applications, are presently under active investigation. Demonstrated applications include fixation of chondrocytes [63] and osteoblasts [64].

Prolamine is a biodegradable protein utilized as a viscous gel [65]. It is amino acid alcohol which polymerizes into a solid compound in the presence of water. It has been used effectively for intravascular arterial occlusion prior to tumor resection [65] and for pancreatic duct occlusion [66] at the time of transplantation. Although used clinically in Europe, it is not approved for use in the United States.

Transforming growth factor beta (TGF-$\beta$) has a chemotactic effect on fibroblasts and stimulates them to produce an extracellular matrix including collagen [67]. Thus, it promotes earlier fibrosis and its effects are evident within four days. It was originally identified in neoplastic cells but can be found in platelets, placenta, and kidney [67]. This agent has been used clinically to promote the healing of retinal tears [68] and is also under further development.

## CONCLUSION

Thus, a spectrum of surgical adhesives exists from the mature, well-developed agents with a large number of established clinical uses, to agents that are early in their developmental stages. Clearly, no effective "glue" is commercially available to the American surgeon today. However, progress is being made in the effort to make safe and effective surgical adhesives widely and easily available at reasonable costs in this country. The development of surgical adhesives remains an exciting and challenging field of clinical research. Further significant progress can be expected.

## REFERENCES

1. Ardis, A. U.S. patent 2,467,927, 1949.
2. Coover, H., Joyner, F. , Shearer, N., et al. Chemistry performance of cyanoacrylate adhesives. *J. Soc. Plas. Surg. Eng.*, 15:5–6, 1959.
3. Watson, D. R. Maguda, T. A. An experimental study for closure of tympanic membrane perforations with fascia and an adhesive. *South. Med. J.*, 58:844–847, 1965.
4. Dean, B. S. Krenzelok, E. P. Cyanoacrylate and corneal abrasion. *Clinical Toxicology*, 27:169–172, 1989.
5. Toriumi, D. M., Taslan, W. F., Friedman, M., Tardy, M. E. Histotoxicity of cyanoacrylate tissue adhesives: A comparison study. *Arch. Otolaryngol. Head and Neck Surg.*, 116:545–550, 1990.
6. Ellis, D. A. F., Shaikh, A. The ideal tissue adhesive in facial and plastic and reconstructive surgery. *J. Otolaryn.*, 19:68–72, 1990.
7. Papaptheofanis, F. J. Cytotoxicity of alkyl-2-cyanoacrylate adhesives. *J. Biomed. Mat. Res.*, 23:661–668, 1989.
8. Papatheofanis, F. J. Prothrombotic cytotoxicity of cyanoacrylate tissue adhesive. *J. Surg. Res.*, 47:309–312, 1989.
9. Samson, D., Marshall, D. Carcinogenic potential of isobutyl-2-cyanoacrylate. *J. Neurosurg.*, 65:571–572, 1986.
10. Brothers, M. F., Kaufman, J. C. E., Fox, A. J., Deveikis, J. P. *n*-Butyl 2-cyanoacrylate–substitute for IBCA an interventional neuroradiology: Histopathologic and polymerization time studies. *AJNR*, 10:777–786, 1989.
11. Kamer, F. M., Joseph, J. H. Histoacryl: Its use in aesthetic facial plastic surgery. *Arch. Otolaryngol. Head and Neck Surg.*, 115:193–197, 1989.
12. Shuber, J. Transcervical sterilization with use of methyl-2-cyanoacrylate and a newer delivery system (the FEMCEPT device). *Am. J. Obstet. Gynecol.*, 160:887–889, 1989.
13. Watson, D. P. Use of cyanoacrylate tissue adhesive for closing facial lacerations in children. *Br. Med. J.*, 299:1014, 1989.
14. Diamond, J. P. Temporary tarsorrhaphy with cyanoacrylate adhesive for seventh-nerve palsy. *The Lancet*, 335:1039, 1990.
15. McCabe, M. J. Use of histoacryl tissue adhesive to manage an avulsed tooth. *Br. Med. J.*, 301:20–21, 1990.
16. Adoni, A., Anteby, E. The use of histoacryl for episiotomy repair. *Br. J. Obstet. Gyn.*, 98:476–478, 1991.
17. Wood, R. E., Lacey, S. R., Azizkhan, R. G. Endoscopic management of large

postresection bronchopleural fistulae with methacrylate adhesive (super glue). *J. Ped. Surg.*, 27:201–202, 1992.

18. Berthelsen, B., Lofgren, J., Svendsen, P. Embolization of cerebral arteriovenous malformations with bucrylate: Experience in a first series of 29 patients. *Acta Radiologica,* 31:13–21, 1991.
19. Gilbert, C. E., Grierson, M., McLeod, D. Retinal patching–A new approach to the management of selected retinal breaks. *Eye,* 3:19–26, 1989.
20. Sheta, S. M., Hilda, T., McCuen, B. W. Cyanoacrylate tissue adhesive in the management of recurrent retinal detachment caused by macular hold. *Am. J. Ophthal.*, 109:28–32, 1989.
21. Papatheofanis, F. J. Surgical repair of rabbit tibia osteotomy using isobutyl-2-cyanoacrylate. *Arch. Orthop. Trauma Surg.*, 108:236–237, 1989.
22. Cavanaugh, T. B., Gottsch, J. D. Infectious keratitis and cyanoacrylate adhesive. *Am. J. Ophthal.*, 111:466–472, 1991.
23. Leahey, A. B., Gottsch, J. D. Sympblepharon associated with cyanoacrylate tissue adhesive. *Arch. Ophthalmol.*, 111:168, 1993.
24. Bergel, S. Uber wirkungen des fibrins. *Dtsch. Med. Wochenschr.*, 35:633, 1909.
25. Young, J. Z., Medawar, P. B. Fibrin suture of peripheral nerves. *Lancet,* 275:126–132, 1940.
26. Cronkite, E. P., Lozner, E. L., Deaver, J. Use of thrombin and fibrinogen in skin grafting. *J. Am. Med. Assoc.*, 124:976–978, 1944.
27. Matras, H., Dings, H. P., Manoli, B., et al. 1972. Zur nachtlosen interfaszikularen nerventransplantation im tierexperiment. *Wein. Med. Wochenschr.*, 122:517–523, 1972.
28. Spotnitz, W. D., Mintz, P. D., Avery, N., Bithell, T. C., Kaul, S., Nolan, S. P. Fibrin glue from stored human plasma: An inexpensive and efficient method for local blood bank preparation. *Am. Surg.*, 53:460–464, 1987.
29. Gestring, G. F., Lerner, R. Autologous fibrinogen for tissue-adhesion, hemostasis, and embolization. *Vasc. Surg.*, 17:294–304, 1983.
30. Siedentop, K. H., Harris, D. M., Sanchez, B. Autologous fibrin tissue adhesive. *Laryngoscope,* 95:1074–1076, 1985.
31. Kjaergard, H. K., Weis-Fogh, U., Sorensen, H., Thiis, J., Rygg, I. Autologous fibrin glue preparation and clinical use in thoracic surgery. *Eur. J. Cardiothorac. Surg.*, 6:52–54, 1992.
32. Nicholas, J. M., Dulchavsky, S. A. Successful use of autologous fibrin gel in traumatic bronchopleural fistula: A case report. *J. Trauma,* 32:87–88, 1992.
33. Oz, M. C., Jeevanadam, V., Smith, C. R., Williams, M. R., Kaynar, A. M., Frank, R. A., Mosca, R., Reiss, R. F., Rose, E. A. Autologous fibrin glue from intraoperatively collected platelet-rich plasma. *Ann. Thorac. Surg.*, 53:530–531, 1992.
34. Kjaergard, H. D., Weis-Fogh, U. S., Thiis, J. J. Preparation of autologous fibrin glue from pericardial blood. *Ann. Thorac. Surg.*, 55:543–544, 1993.
35. Seelich, T. Inactivation of pathogens, e.g., viruses, in tissue adhesive containing factor XIII and fibrinogen by heating in dry state in absence of oxygen. European Patent 85890227.

36. Horowitz, M. S., Rooks, C., Horowitz, B., Hilgartner, M. W. Virus safety of solvent/detergent-treated antihemophilic factor concentrate. *Lancet,* 8604:186–188, 1988.
37. Lerner, R., Birnus, N. S. Current status of surgical adhesives. *J. Surg. Res.,* 48:165–181, 1990.
38. Sierra, D. H. Fibrin sealant adhesive systems: A review of their chemistry, material properties and clinical applications. *J. Biomat. App.,* 7:309–352, 1993.
39. Rapaport, I. S., Zivelin, A., Minow, R. A., Huner, C. S., Donnelly, K. Clinical significance of antibodies to bovine and human thrombin and factor V after surgical use of bovine thrombin. *Am. J. Clin. Pathol.,* 97:84–91, 1992.
40. Berruyer, M., Amiral, J., Ffrench, P., Belleville, J., Bastien, O., Clerc, J., Kassir, A., Estanove, S., Dechavanne, M. Immunization by bovine thrombin used with fibrin glue during cardiovascular operations: Development of thrombin and factor V inhibitors. *J. Thorac. Cardiovasc. Surg.,* 105:892–897, 1993.
41. Kanchuger, M. S., Eide, T. R., Mancke, G. R., Hartman, A., Poppers, P. J. The hemodynamic effects of topical fibrin glue during cardia operations. *J. Cardiothorac. Anesth.,* 3:745–747, 1989.
42. Milde, L. N. An anaphylactic reaction to fibrin glue. *Anesth. Analg.,* 69:684–686, 1989.
43. Pipan, C. M., Glasheen, W. P., Matthew, T. L., Gonias, S. L., Hwang, L. J., Jane, J. A., Spotnitz, W. D. Effects of antifibrinolytic agents on the life span of fibrin sealant. *J. Surg. Res.,* 53:402–407, 1992.
44. Byrne, D. J., Hardy, J., Wood, R. A., McIntosh, B., Cuschieri, A. Effect of fibrin glues on the mechanical properties of healing wounds. *Br. J. Surg.,* 78:841–843, 1991.
45. Redl, H., Schlag, G., Stanek, G., Hirschl, A., Seelick, T. In vitro properties of mixtures of fibrin seal and antibiotics. *Biomaterials,* 4:29–32, 1983.
46. Kram, H. B., Bansul, M., Timberlake, O., et al. Antibacterial effects of fibrin glue on fibrin glue-antibiotic mixtures. *Trans. Soc. Biomat.,* 12:164, 1989.
47. Greco, F., DePalma, L., Spagnolo, N., Rossi, A., Specchia, N., Gigante, A. Fibrin-antibiotic mixtures: An in vitro study assessing the possibility of using a biological carrier for local drug delivery. *J. Biomed. Mat. Res.,* 25:39–51, 1991.
48. Sugitachi, A., Shindo, T., Kido, T., Kawahara, T. Bioadhesiochemo-(BAC)-therapy. *Proc. Amer. Assoc. Cancer Res.,* 33:216, 1992.
49. Matthew, T. L., Spotnitz, W. D., Kron, I. L., Daniel, T. M., Tribble, C. G., Nolan, S. P. Four years' experience with fibrin sealant in thoracic and cardiovascular surgery. *Ann. Thorac. Surg.,* 50:40–44, 1990.
50. Shaffrey, C. I., Spotnitz, W. D., Shaffrey, M. E., Jane, J. A. Neurosurgical applications of fibrin glue: Augmentation of dural closure in 134 patients. *Neurosurgery,* 26:207–210, 1990.
51. Straindl, O. Tissue adhesion with highly concentrated human fibrinogen in otolaryngology. *Ann. Otol. Rhinol. Laryngol.,* 88:413–418, 1979.
52. Lagoutte, F. M., Gauthier, L., Comte, P. R. A fibrin sealant for perforated and preperforated corneal ulcers. *Br. J. Ophthalmol.,* 73:757–761, 1989.
53. Stuart, J. D., Kenney, J. G., Lettieri, J., Spotnitz, W., Baker, J. Application of single donor fibrin glue to burns. *J. Burn Care Rehab.,* 9:619–622, 1988.

54. Baker, J. W., Spotnitz, W. D., Nolan, S. P. A technique for spray application of fibrin glue during cardiac operations. *Ann. Thorac. Surg.*, 43:564–565, 1987.
55. Bachet, J., Goudot, B., Teodori, G., Brodaty, D., Dubois, C., De Lentdecker, P H., Guilmet, D. Surgery of type a acute aortic dissection with gelatin-resorcine-formol biological glue: A twelve year experience. *J. Cardiovasc. Surg.*, 31:263–273, 1990.
56. Guilmet, D., Bachet, J., Goudot, B., Laurian, C., Gigou, F., Bical, O., Barbagelatta, M. Use of biologic glue in acute aortic dissection. A new surgical technique. Preliminary clinical results. *J. Thorac. Cardiovasc. Surg.*, 77:516–521, 1979.
57. Portoghese, M., Acar, C., Jebara, V., Chachques, J. C., Fontaliran, F., Deloche, A., Carpentier, A. Alterations de la paroi vasculaire dues aux colles chirurgicales: Etude experimentale. *La Presse Medicale,* 21:1154–1156, 1992.
58. Fabiani, J. N., Jebara, V. A., Deloche, A., Stephan, Y., Carpentier, A. Use of surgical glue without replacement in the treatment of type a aortic dissection. *Circulation,* 80:264–268, 1989.
59. Cooper, C. W., Grode, G. A., Falb, R. D. The chemistry of bonding: Alternative approaches to adhesive joining of tissue. In: *Tissue Adhesives in Surgery,* T. Matsumoto, ed. Medical Examination Publishing Co., Inc., New York, 1972.
60. Waite, J. H. The formation of mussel byssus: Anatomy of a natural manufacturing process. In: *Structure, Cellular Synthesis and Assembly of Biopolymers,* S. T. Case, ed. Springer-Verlag, New York, pp. 27–54, 1992.
61. Laursen, R. A. Reflection on the structure of mussel adhesive protein. In: *Structure, Cellular Synthesis and Assembly of Biopolymers,* S. T. Case, ed. New York: Springer-Verlag, pp. 55–74, 1992.
62. Liggett, P. E., Cano, M., Robin, J. B., Green, R. L., Lean, J. S. Intravitreal biocompatibility of mussel adhesive protein. A preliminary study. *Retina,* 10:144–147, 1990.
63. Pitman, M. I., Menche, D., Song, E. K., Ben-Yishay, A., Gilbert, D., Grande, D. A. The use of adhesives in chondrocyte transplantation surgery: In vivo studies. *Bulletin of the Hospital for Joint Diseases Orthopaedic Institute,* 49:213–221, 1989.
64. Fulkerson, J. P., Norton, L. A., Gronowicz, G., Picciano, P., Massicotte, J. M., Nissen, C. W. Attachment of epiphyseal cartilage cells and 17/28 rat osteosarcoma osteoblasts using mussel adhesive protein. *J. Orthop. Res.*, 8:793–798, 1990.
65. Pigott, J. P., Donovan, D. L., Fink, J. A., Sharp, W. V. Angioscope-assisted occlusion of venous tributaries with prolamine in in situ femoropopliteal by-pass: Preliminary results of canine experiments. *J. Vasc. Surg.*, 9:704–709, 1989.
66. Torino, F., Gil, O., Garaycoechea, M., Garcia, H., Casavilla, A., Shenk, C., Hojman, D. Pancreatic duct occlusion in the management of acute necrotizing pancreatitis in a canine model. *Mount Sinai Journal of Medicine,* 56:79–82, 1989.
67. Sporn, M. B., Roberts, A. B., Wakefield, L. M., et al. Some recent advances in the chemistry and biology of transforming growth factor-beta. *J. Cell. Biol.*, 105:1039–1045, 1987.
68. Smiddy, W. E., Glaser, B. M., Green, W. R., Connor, T. B., Roberts, A. B., Lucas, R., Sporn, M. B. Transforming growth factor beta. *Arch. Ophthalmol.*, 107:577–580, 1989.

# *Chapter 2: Commercial Pooled-Source Fibrin Sealant*

M. J. MacPHEE

## INTRODUCTION

The use of adhesives and sealants in medical applications may date back as far as 4000 years [1]. Throughout history scientists and healers have strived to improve the technology, and today's sutures and sealants/adhesives are both effective and reliable. Nevertheless, there are situations in which sutures and chemical adhesives may fail to perform adequately or may introduce unwanted side effects due to their inherent incompatibility with the natural processes of wound healing and tissue regeneration that are active in the tissue into which they must be placed [2]. One sealant/adhesive that has undergone significant development in the twentieth century is fibrin. This natural, hemostatic sealant/adhesive is produced by the body at the site of any vascular injury and, thus, it has the advantage of being not only effective, but also being compatible with natural healing and regenerative processes.

The first correct description of the roles of fibrin, thrombin, and $Ca^{2+}$ in the process of blood clotting was in 1905 by Morawitz. In 1909, Bergel reported the hemostatic effects of powdered fibrin [3]. As has often been the case, it was war that provided the impetus for the next development in the therapeutic application of fibrin. Faced with large numbers of casualties suffering severe blood loss, surgeons in World War I began to use sheets of fibrin during surgery for the treatment of injuries. This approach, pioneered by Grey [4], met with some success. In 1940 Young and Medawar used a combination of plasma and thrombin during surgery to seal nerves. Improvements in fibrinogen remained incremental with the trend being toward a more purified set of components. In 1944 Cronkite et al. were the first to combine purified fibrinogen and thrombin in clinical use [5]. In 1972, Matras et al. [6] used a concentrated fibrinogen in combination with purified

***Table 2.1.*** *Current producers of pooled commercial fibrin sealant (worldwide).*

| Company | Product | Fibrinogen | Thrombin | Viral Inactivation |
|---|---|---|---|---|
| Immuno AG | Tisseel® | Human | Bovine/Human | Heat |
| Behringwerke AG | Beriplast™ | Human | Bovine | Heat |
| CRTS-Lille (LFB) | Biocol™ | Human | Bovine | S-D |
| Kaketsuken | Bolheal™ | Human | Human | Heat |

Factor XIII and an antiprotease to seal nerve endings. The experience with these substances made it clear that an effective, consistent, and controllable formulation would find numerous applications, including their use to prevent blood and fluid loss from traumatic injuries and burns as well as a biocompatible adhesive in plastic or reconstructive surgery.

These "homemade" fibrin-based adhesives and hemostatic treatments remained the state of the art until the 1980s when commercial products prepared from pooled plasma became available, first in Europe and then in Canada and Japan. Current producers of these products are listed in Table 2.1. These products gained rapid acceptance, and their use has been extended to almost all fields of surgery.

## PRODUCTION ISSUES

Pooled fibrinogen-thrombin products are frequently referred to as "fibrin glue" or "fibrin sealant." For the purpose of this chapter the latter term will be used. Fibrin sealant prepared from plasma pooled from a large number of donors has several advantages over preparations made using cryoprecipitate plasma from a single donor (hereafter referred to as "cryo"). The most important of these include product consistency, availability, purity, and cost. Product consistency is a vital concern. Variation in the concentrations of total protein, fibrinogen, Factor XIII, and proteolytic activity in single-donor preparations may lead to uncertainty regarding the reliability of cryo in surgical applications.

Commercial pooled products are subject to strictly defined product specifications regarding these and other critical components. They may be purchased in advance and kept in stock in emergency rooms, surgical suites, and hospital pharmacies. While cryo may be produced in advance and stored, it places a significantly greater burden on each facility to obtain and screen donors, and prepare and store the cryo rather than ordering it from a manufacturer. Additionally, while cryo must be thawed prior to use, commercial products are generally lyophilized and require little time and attention to prepare for use. These are factors that may be important in treating critically ill patients. Finally, the number of people required to produce and prepare cryo may make cost a consideration and limit its use to those institutions with sufficient infrastructure to support its production [7].

## PRODUCT SAFETY

The major challenges to producers of pooled fibrin sealant products are product safety, product consistency, regulatory approval, product availability, and ease of use. In regard to the issue of product safety the risk of viral transmission remains the major concern. There are several crucial steps in manufacture that can be utilized to minimize the risk of disease transmission. The first is donor screening. An intensive questioning of potential donors combined with testing for exposure to pathogens can significantly reduce the chances that plasma-containing pathogens may enter the production process.

The second critical step is inactivation of potential viral pathogens. Currently, three processes are generally recognized as being effective in inactivating virus in plasma: heat inactivation, solvent/detergent treatment, and ultrafiltration. Each of these methods has advantages when applied to the treatment of fibrinogen-containing preparations and a detailed discussion of them is beyond the scope of this chapter. It is interesting to note that the first manufacturer of pooled-fibrin sealant in Europe utilized heat treatment, while the newest manufacturer uses the solvent/detergent method.

The final step in ensuring product safety is postproduction testing. This may include tests for specific pathogens that may have escaped inactivation during manufacture.

Another safety consideration relates to the source of the components used in the fibrin sealant. There are two potential concerns. They both relate to the use of nonhuman source materials, chiefly in the form of bovine thrombin or aprotinin. The use of these nonhuman products may result in anaphylactic reactions in patients sensitive to them. The use of bovine thrombin has also been associated with a few cases of autoantibody generation against the patient's own thrombin, resulting in increased clotting times [8].

An additional concern related to using bovine-derived products is the possible transmission of bovine spongioform encephalopathy (BSE). BSE is believed to be caused by the same transmissible agent that causes scrapie in sheep. This agent is believed to have infected cattle through feed that contained sheep by-products. The ability of this disease to be transmitted across species has led to concern that bovine-derived products from infected cattle might be capable of passing the disease on to patients. This issue has resulted in several countries placing restrictions on bovine-derived products from countries where BSE is now established.

Issues regarding product consistency are managed by the use of plasma pooled from large numbers of donors, the application of appropriate product specifications for the final product, consistent manufacturing methods, and rigorous postmanufacturing quality-control testing. Product availability is obviously dependent upon correct forecasting of demand for the product and by securing access to a sufficiently large number of healthy plasma donors to prevent shortfalls in the supply of input material.

## APPLICATION OF FIBRIN SEALANTS

Ease of use of the final product is largely associated with two procedures: reconstitution and application. Reconstitution of fibrin-sealant products may be difficult owing to the relatively high concentration of fibrinogen in the reconstituted liquid. In the past this has resulted in the need for complicated and potentially expensive warming/mixing devices as well as training in their use. Better product formulation may reduce the time required for reconstitution, and possibly eliminate the need for ancillary warming/mixing devices.

Ease of application may be maximized by providing delivery devices that are simple to load and operate, and that meet the needs of the practitioner applying the fibrin sealant. A number of delivery systems have been developed for applying the material directly to a site as a small droplet or bead, for delivery through cannulas, and for application as a spray to cover large areas [2].

Various manufacturers supply devices to fill these needs with each design having particular advantages. Ordinarily the manufacturer of the fibrin sealant will supply several different delivery devices for different procedures, providing the practitioner the opportunity to choose the appropriate applicator. In choosing a design, a manufacturer must take care to select only that which is effective and easy to use.

## AVAILABILITY OF COMMERCIAL PRODUCTS

While commercial pooled fibrin sealants have been available in Europe

***Table 2.2.*** *Pooled fibrin sealant: organizations pursuing the U.S. market.*

| Organization | Composition | Viral Inactivation | Stage |
|---|---|---|---|
| Alpha Therapeutics | Human | S-D[b] | Preclinical |
| ARC[a] | Human | S-D/Heat/Filtration | Clinical trials |
| Baxter-Hyland | Human | S-D/Heat/Filtration | Clinical trials |
| Haemacure | Human | S-D/Heat/Filtration | Preclinical |
| Immuno AG | Human/Bovine | Heat | Clinical trials |
| NY Blood Center/ Melville Biologics | Human | S-D/UV-C[c] | Preclinical |

[a]ARC = American Red Cross.
[b]S-D = Solvent-Detergent.
[c]UV-C = Ultraviolet light, waveband C.

and Canada for over a decade, there is currently no licensed producer in the United States. The reasons for this are too complex for discussion at this time, but it must be kept in mind that these products are subject to the same regulatory approval processes as other plasma derivatives. Careful attention must be paid to the design and analysis of clinical trials, along with appropriate manufacturing controls in order to succeed with licensure.

At the time this was written, the author was able to identify seven organizations developing pooled fibrin-sealant products in the United States (subject to regulatory approval by the FDA). These are shown in Table 2.2. This information was correct at the time of writing, but it must be kept in mind that formulations, viral-inactivation methods, and research and development plans may change without notice. Readers wishing precise information on a product are advised to contact these organizations for details.

## CONCLUSION

In conclusion, scientists have found many uses for fibrinogen-based adhesive/hemostatic products in modern surgical techniques. These products have well-established safety records in Europe and Canada, and several organizations are attempting to develop products for licensure in the United States. To reach this goal numerous challenges exist in assuring product safety, efficacy, consistency, and availability. Successful products should have a profound effect upon many surgical procedures.

## REFERENCES


1. Saltz, R., Sierra, D., Feldman, D., Bartczak-Saltz, M., Dimick, A., Vasconez, L. O. Experimental and clinical applications of fibrin glue. *Plast. Reconstr. Surg.*, 88:1005, 1991.
2. Sierra, D. Fibrin sealant adhesive systems: A review of their chemistry, material properties and clinical applications. *J. Biomater. Appl.*, 7:309, 1991.
3. Bergel, S. Uber wirkungen des fibrins. *Dtsch. Med. Wochenschr.*, 35:633, 1909.
4. Grey, E. Fibrin as a hemostatic in cerebral surgery. *Surg. Gynecol. Obstet.*, 21:452, 1915.
5. Cronkite, E., Lozner, E., Deaver, J. Use of thrombin and fibrinogen in skin grafting. *JAMA*, 124:976, 1944.
6. Matras, H., Dinges, H., Manoli, B. Zur nachtlosen interfaszikularen nerventransplantation im tierexperiment. *Wien. Med. Woschtr.*, 122:517, 1972.
7. Casali, B., Rodeghiero, F., Tosetto, A., Palmieri, B., Immovilli, R., Ghedini, C., Rivasi, P. Fibrin glue from single-donation autologous plasmapheresis. *Transfusion*, 32:641, 1992.
8. Rapaport, S., Zivelin, A., Minow, R., Hunter, C., Donnelly, K. Clinical significance of antibodies to bovine and human thrombin and factor V after surgical use of bovine thrombin. *Amer. J. Clin. Path.*, 97:84, 1992.

# *Chapter 3: Mussel Adhesive Protein*

K. GREEN

## INTRODUCTION

Mussel adhesive protein (MAP) is secreted by a gland of the marine mollusk *Mytilus edulis* and other bivalves. It serves to attach the mollusk to rocks or other substrates in the turbulent tidal zones, thereby demonstrating its powerful adhesive properties. The natural product is a protein of 120K dalton molecular weight that contains a repeated decapeptide rich in lysine, hydroxylated amino acids, and dopa [1–5]. This material, which cures rapidly upon contact with water, was patented by Waite.

MAP has been shown to serve as an enhancer of cell attachment to plastic in tissue culture, including cells derived from ocular tissues [6,7]. Furthermore, it has been proposed as an adhesive in the application of shaped portions of stroma and synthetic materials to the anterior surface of the cornea in order to alter its refractive power (epikeratoplasty) [8]. The ability of MAP to enhance cell attachment severalfold to plastic tissue culture dishes also suggests the possible use of this adhesive as a coating of the anterior stromal surface in order to provide a platform upon which epithelial regrowth could occur in disorders such as recurrent epithelial erosion, diabetes, and corneal ulcers [6,7]. This would take advantage of the cellular adhesion properties of the adhesive when used in this manner.

## MATERIALS AND METHODS

Following the identification of the chemical constituents of MAP, synthetic polymers were manufactured that were branch copolymers with a free-amine-rich linear backbone onto which were grafted variations of the natural decapeptide. All of these latter compounds are the subject of a patent by Bio-Polymers [9]. While the tissue culture derivative has entered the commercial market (Cell-Tak, Collaborative Research Incorporated, Biomedical Products Division, Bedford, MA), the remaining materials are currently "on hold" due to the loss of venture capital funding in 1992.

A large number of compounds have been tested for their ocular toxicity. This contribution provides a summary of the data accumulated to date on the ocular toxicity of those compounds. Specific data are not presented, but rather, generalizations of the total ocular reaction are presented. Although the ideal test condition for such an adhesive would be during a surgical procedure, it is difficult to separate the varying factors that would coexist following such treatment and isolate those changes induced only by the adhesive. It was decided, therefore, to perform standard ocular toxicity testing in adult albino rabbits with delivery of material to one of two sites. All tests were performed in a masked manner with the investigator being unaware of the chemical nature of the test materials. Each substance or mixture was identified only by code.

The primary site of injection for toxicity, since the majority of the projected use of the material would be outside the globe, was an intrastromal site, with other injections being made intracamerally (into the anterior chamber of the eye). The latter injections were performed using an atraumatic technique developed in this laboratory [10–12]. A 30-gauge needle attached to a Gilmont microsyringe was inserted subepithelially for 2 to 3 mm before being pushed through the stroma into the anterior chamber. After appropriate volume injection, the needle was withdrawn to the sub-epithelial location and about thirty seconds were allowed for the corneal stroma to swell before needle removal [13]. This procedure results in a leakproof seal with no loss of aqueous humor and, thus, no disturbance to the eye. For intrastromal injections the needle tip is placed within the stroma and can be immediately withdrawn from the cornea after injection. The volume of the injections in the majority of experiments was 13 $\mu$L, with appropriate adjustments of volumes of individual compounds to sum to 13 $\mu$L. All injections were performed only after systemic anesthesia with xylazine (10 mg) and ketamine (100 mg) given intramuscularly. The contralateral eye received an injection of balanced salt solution (BSS; Alcon, Fort Worth, TX) in the same location as the ipsilateral eye.

The ocular tissue reactions were scored using the Draize scale for conjunctival chemosis and hyperemia, iritis, anterior chamber cell and flare, hyperemia of the iris, the degree and area of corneal edema. Any lens changes were scored on a 0 to 4+ scale (i.e.: 0, 0+, 1, 1+. . .). Eyes were examined by slit-lamp biomicroscope. Corneal thickness was also measured using a pachometer attachment to a Haag-Streit 900 slit lamp. Measurements and observations were made on day 0 (prior to injection), day 1, day

2, day 3 and day 7. After the day 7 readings, the rabbits were sacrificed with an intravenous overdose of sodium pentobarbital and anterior segments of eyes were removed and fixed in 10% formalin prior to embedding in paraffin. Tissue blocks were sectioned 8 $\mu$m thick and stained with hematotoxylin and eosin. Sections were examined with a Zeiss photomicroscope. All experiments were conducted with adherence to the Regulations on the Use of Animals in Research approved by ARVO and the guidelines of the Medical College of Georgia Committee on Animal Use in Research and Education.

## RESULTS

The ocular toxicity data summaries for intracameral injections are given in Table 3.1, and summaries for intrastromal injections are given in Table 3.2; these results are based on two to six observations per compound. Responses were called either "normal" or "no response" when an ocular reaction was absent. A small response (1+) usually involved a short duration (twenty-four hours) conjunctival hyperemia of 0+ to 1 grade that was associated with a small (i.e., <50 $\mu$m) increase in corneal thickness. A moderate response (2+) was indicative of a greater conjunctival reaction (1+ to 2+ hyperemia) sometimes lasting up to forty-eight hours with some intraocular cells and flare and an increase in corneal thickness of about 100 $\mu$m with iris hyperemia. A significant or large response (3+) usually included conjunctival hyperemia of at least forty-eight to seventy-two hours duration, with corneal thickness involvement of about a 100 to 250 $\mu$m increase in thickness. Recovery was either complete or partially complete by seven days. A large (4+) response was the most pronounced response that involved conjunctival hyperemia of about 2 to 2+, and in a considerable number of cells and flare in the anterior chamber sometimes sufficient to obliterate viewing of the iris. In some cases recovery occurred but frequently the inflammatory reaction lasted for seven days, albeit decreasing in intensity with time.

No control eye, whether after intrastromal or intracameral injection of BSS, showed any reaction; in a rare instance a 0+ conjunctival hyperemia was seen at twenty-four hours. Apart from a few occurrences these eyes were quiet and no toxicity occurred. Changes from normal, therefore, represented toxicity induced by chemical rather than mechanical irritation.

There was a significant difference between the responses to the same adhesive material when injected at the two different sites. Most compounds injected into the anterior chamber induced some degree of intraocular inflammation and/or corneal swelling. This response indicated a marked

***Table 3.1.*** *Intraocular response after injection of synthetic adhesives into the anterior chamber.*

| **Intracameral Injections:** | | |
|---|---|---|
| A | Nonapeptide, two dopa residues | No response |
| B | Forty residue peptide, eight dopa residues on polylysine-tyrosine | Significant (+ + +) response. Effects still present but less at seven days |
| B2 | B plus free amine cross-linker: bis(sulfosuccinimidyl) suberate | Large (+ + + +) immediate response. Cleared by seven days |
| C | Decapeptide, two dopa residues on polylysine-alanine | Minor response |
| C2 | C plus free amine cross-linker | Small immediate response (+) |
| D | Nonapeptide, two dopa residues on polyallylamine | Moderate immediate response (+ +) |
| D2 | D plus cross-linker | Moderate immediate response (+ +) |
| E | Nonapeptide, two dopa residues on polylysine | Large response (+ + +) |
| E2 | E plus cross-linker | Large response (+ + +) |
| F | Nonapeptide, two dopa residues on polylysine | Large response (+ + + +) with slow recovery |
| F2 | F plus cross-linker | Large response (+ + + +) with slow recovery |
| G | Nonapeptide, one dopa residue on polyallylamine | Significant (+ +) to large (+ + + +) response |
| G2 | G plus cross-linker | Large response (+ + +); recovery by seventy-two hours with some cross-linkers, no recovery at seven days with others. Normal to moderate response; full recovery by 48 hours |

Different cross-linkers gave different responses.

toxic reaction that involved the iris and the infiltration of inflammatory cells either locally or from the systemic circulation. Further, the occurrence of corneal swelling indicated a toxic reaction of the corneal endothelium.

Three of the materials, a nonapeptide with two dopa residues (compound A) and a decapeptide with two dopa residues on polylysine-alanine (compound C), either alone or admixed with cross-linker (compound C2), demonstrated the least ocular toxicity after intracameral injection. The other compounds (D, D2) caused only a moderate immediate response that recovered very quickly (i.e., by forty-eight hours). At least some of the compounds, therefore, did not evoke a serious toxicological response and would be predicted to have minimal effects in humans.

Histopathology of an inflamed eye after intracameral injection frequently revealed proteinaceous material in the anterior chamber with inflammatory cells involving both the iris and aqueous humor. The inflammation should have at least a seven-day duration. This is a necessary factor since all experiments ran for seven days and obviously substantial recovery of the normal condition could and often did occur in the time before removal of tissues for histological assessment. The ciliary processes, located on the surface of the iris, that play a significant role in aqueous humor formation were often swollen and contained epithelial cysts. This response is typical of a reaction to toxic substances. In addition, iris vessels are often dilated again indicating an inflammatory response. In several cases the material injected could be observed as a flocculent mass in the anterior chamber.

Injections into the stroma appeared to offer some protection to the eye when compared to intracameral injections of the same material. Intrastromal injections evoked less overall ocular toxicity with the most often noted reaction being no observable responses. Presumably the marked reduction in response to the same volume of material that induced large responses when injected into the anterior chamber was caused by the location of the compound in the stroma. Not only does this site physically separate the stroma environment from the aqueous humor, but also, because the material cures rapidly in the stroma, there is a reduced opportunity for

***Table 3.2.*** *Ocular toxicity after injection of synthetic adhesives into the corneal stroma.*

| **Intrastromal Injections:** | | |
|---|---|---|
| (The identification system is the same as that for intracameral injections.) | | |
| D2 | Nonapeptide, two dopa residues on a polyallylamine plus cross-linker | Normal |
| E | Nonapeptide, one dopa residue on polylysine | Large response (+ + + +); some recovery at seven days |
| E1 | E but different manufacturing process | Normal |
| E2 | E plus cross-linker | Large response (+ + +); some recovery at seven days |
| F | Nonapeptide, two dopa residues on polylysine | Normal |
| G | Nonapeptide, one dopa residue on polyallylamine | Small (+) to no response |
| G | G with different manufacturing process | Normal |
| G | G plus cross-linker | Normal |
| H | MAP | Normal |
| | Cross-linkers | Normal to moderate (+ +) response; when present continued to seven days |

In many cases material could be visualized in the stroma as an elliptical "veil" lying between corneal lamellae.

further penetration into other ocular compartments. Where intraocular toxicity exists, this indicates that some component of the material can escape its intrastromal location and enter the anterior chamber. Several compounds (Table 3.2) showed little or no toxicity. These were D2, E1, F, G, G1, G2 and H. D2 and G2 included the presence of a free-amine cross-linker. The only common chemical that induced no or minimal toxicity at either location was D2 (and presumably D, although the latter was only tested intracamerally).

Histopathology of corneas after intrastromal injection was usually normal, especially where no toxic reaction occurred. Where an involvement occurred, macrophages were present at or near the injected material. The latter could often be identified between lamellae within the cornea as a thick layer of crystalline or cellophane-like material. In most cases where involvement occurred, there was also a change in the appearance of the keratocytes (cells that manufacture the glycoprotein matrix of the corneal stroma) in the stroma that took on the appearance of overreactive fibroblasts.

## DISCUSSION

The potential of these bioadhesives lies in their rapid curing and vigorous adhesive properties. The ability of MAP to act as a strong biological adhesive in freshly isolated ocular tissues offers potential use in many circumstances. Both retina and Descemet's membrane become strongly attached to either, similar to tissue or plastic [6]. The adhesive power of these tissue glues suggests that they could be used under a variety of conditions both intraocularly and extraocularly. Extraocular use includes use as a material for the closure of lesions (incisions after intraocular surgery–accidental cuts in the eye associated with ocular trauma) and use as a surface material for coating the anterior surface of the cornea to allow better regrowth of corneal epithelium (recurrent corneal erosions; diabetes, where epithelial growth is stunted; corneal ulcers where epithelial loss contributes to progression of the disorder). Intraocular use would involve readherence of the retina to the underlying tissues after retinal detachment, or reattachment of the iris root if a cyclodialysis cleft is present between the iris and more peripheral ocular tissues.

Regardless of the potential location of the materials in or on the eye, we have previously shown [14] that polymerized MAP offers no barrier to the diffusion of nonelectrolytes that vary in size from insulin (5K daltons molecular weight) to dextran (72K daltons). The permeability of MAP is at least equal to that of the corneal stroma [14]. If MAP offers no barrier to compounds of this size and shape, then no diffusional barrier exists to any molecule of consequence to metabolism. Thus, any cells growing on MAP, when used as a substrate, will have no disruption of essential catabolic or anabolic metabolism.

Where recovery from inflammation and corneal swelling occurs, care must be exercised in interpretation of such an event in the rabbit model. There are two aspects to this phenomenon. The first concerns the degree of inflammation of the rabbit eye to the same dose of stimulant [15 – 19]. The response differential is roughly tenfold, i.e., a 10 $\mu$L drop of a material in the rabbit eye is equivalent to a 100 $\mu$L drop of the same material at an identical concentration in the human eye. The responses noted in the albino rabbit eye, therefore, must be tempered by the consideration that the model shows a large inflammatory response to stimuli [19]. In this respect the rabbit eye is unique, yet it stands as the classical model for the assessment of ocular irritation potential [20 – 25].

The second aspect concerns the recovery of corneal thickness as well as the rate of recovery for intraocular inflammation. The corneal endothelium of the rabbit has extraordinary recovery power. Even destruction by cryoprobe resulting in the loss of endothelial cells over a wide area does not prevent complete recovery within five to seven days [24,25]. The result (after such a destructive procedure) is a cornea that is indistinguishable from normal. However, recovery does not occur in humans because the endothelium does not regrow after destruction of a large area. Smaller area losses of endothelial cells, with no more than ten to fifteen contiguous cells, can be covered again by cells due to cellular expansion, but cellular multiplication and division do not occur. Intraocular inflammation and corneal swelling caused by intraocular placement of the adhesives would appear to induce too much endothelial damage in many cases for recovery in a human endothelium.

The other aspect of recovery, namely that from inflammation, also concerns the relative changes in rabbits and humans. While the initial responses in a rabbit tend to be vigorous compared to the usually lower level of response to the same stimuli in a human, the return to normality occurs with great rapidity in a rabbit whereas an inflammatory reaction induced in a human tends to continue at a lower level for a significant time. In a rabbit, therefore, a violent inflammatory response can occur within twenty-four hours of an insult with complete recovery by seventy-two hours. In a human, by comparison, a far lesser initial response may reduce slightly, but still be present after seven to fourteen days.

All of the above points out that the rabbit eye responses must be viewed from these different perspectives and used as an index for potential human responses. The responses have to be considered against the background of the known differential between the two species in predicting the level of toxicity in the human eye.

The overall use of these bioadhesives as an ocular material has not progressed to clinical trials, but the potential exists for numerous uses in ophthalmology. Based on the present data, the primary use as an externally applied agent would be the easiest goal to achieve. The demonstrated decrease in toxicity when materials are placed intrastromally compared to intracameral injection makes their extraocular use a distinct possibility. Intraocular use, or use under circumstances where direct access to the intraocular environment would be possible, is not yet practical given the compounds tested in these studies. The intraocular use of such materials must await further delineation of those portions of the molecule that induce the toxic reaction. Some compounds, however, seem to possess the necessary characteristics that would allow their intraocular use. The nonapeptide with dopa residues on polyallylamine (compound D or D2) seems to offer a pathway for continued exploration of its use both intra- and extraocularly.

## ACKNOWLEDGEMENTS

These studies were performed between November 1988 and June 1989 and were supported by Bio-Polymers, Inc., Connecticut. I thank Dr. Harry Gossling for his permission to publish this data, and Dr. Christine V. Benedict for her invaluable help in providing the interpretation of the code numbers that were known in my laboratory. Thanks are due to both for their efforts in helping to coordinate laboratory code numbers to chemical structures. Lisa Cheeks provided valuable technical assistance, and Brenda Sheppard provided secretarial assistance.

## REFERENCES

1. Waite, J. H. Evidence for a repeating 3,4-dihydroxyphenylalanine- and hydroxyproline-containing decapeptide in the adhesive protein of the mussel, *Mytilus edulis L. J. Biol. Chem.*, 258:2911–2915, 1983.
2. Benedict, C. V., Waite, J. H. Composition and ultrastructure of the byssus of *Mytilus edulis. J. Morphol.*, 189:261–270, 1986.
3. Waite, J. H. Mussel glue from *Mytilus californiamus Conrad*: A comparative study. *J. Comp. Physiol.*, 156:491–496, 1986.
4. Williams, T., Marumo, K., Waite, J. H., Henkens, R. W. Mussel glue protein has an open configuration. *Arch. Biochem. Biophys.*, 269:415–422, 1989.
5. Waite, J. H., Hansen, D. C., Little, K. T. The glue protein of ribbed mussels (*Geukensia demissa*): A natural adhesive with some features of collagen. *J. Comp. Physiol.*, 159:517–525, 1989.
6. Picciano, P. T., Benedict, C. V. Mussel adhesive protein: A new epithelium tissue adhesive and cell attachment factor. *Invest. Ophthalmol. Vis. Sci.*, 27(suppl):31, 1986.
7. Picciano, P. T., Benedict, C. V. Mussel adhesive protein: A new cell attachment factor. *In Vitro Cell Develop. Biol.*, 22(suppl):24A, 1986.

8. Robin, J. B., Picciano, P., Kusleika, R. S., Salazar, J., Benedict, C. Preliminary evaluation of the use of mussel adhesive protein in experimental keratoplasty. *Arch. Ophthalmol.*, 106:973–977, 1988.
9. Waite, J. H. Decapeptides produced from bioadhesive polyphenolic proteins. U.S. Patent 4,585,585, 1986.
10. Csukas, S., Green, K. Effects of intracameral hydrogen peroxide in the rabbit anterior chamber. *Invest. Ophthalmol. Vis. Sci.*, 29:335–339, 1988.
11. Csukas, S., Costarides, A., Riley, M. V., Green, K. Hydrogen peroxide in the rabbit anterior chamber: Effects on glutathione, and catalase effects on peroxide kinetics. *Curr. Eye Res.*, 6:1395–1402, 1987.
12. Costarides, A. P., Riley, M. V., Green, K. Roles of catalase and the glutathione redox cycle in the regulation of anterior chamber hydrogen peroxide. *Ophthalmic Res.*, 23:284–294, 1991.
13. Friedman, H. H., Green, K. Swelling rate of corneal stroma. *Exp. Eye Res.*, 12:239–250, 1971.
14. Green, K., Berdecia, R., Cheeks, L. Mussel adhesive protein: Permeability characteristics when used as a basement membrane. *Curr. Eye Res.*, 6:835–838, 1987.
15. Griffith, J. F., Nixon, G. A., Bruce, R. D., Reer, P. J., Bannan, E. A. Dose response studies with chemical irritants in the albino rabbit eye as a basis for selecting optimum testing conditions for predicting hazard to the human eye. *Toxicol. Appl. Pharmacol.*, 5:501–513, 1982.
16. Freeberg, F. E., Nixon, G. A., Reer, P. J., Weaver, J. E., Bruce, R. D., Griffith, J. F., Sanders, L. W. Human and rabbit eye responses to chemical insult. *Fundam. Appl. Toxicol.*, 7:626–634, 1986.
17. Freeberg, F. E., Griffith, J. F., Bruce, R. D., Bay, P. H. S. Correlation of animal test methods with human exposure for household products. *J. Toxicol. Cutan. Ocular Toxicol.*, 1:53–64, 1984.
18. Allgood, G. S. Use of animal test data and human experience for determining the ocular irritation potential of shampoos. *J. Toxicol. Cutan. Ocular Toxicol.*, 8:321–326, 1989.
19. Bito, L. Z. Species differences in the responses of the eye to irritation and trauma: A hypothesis of divergence in ocular defense mechanisms, and the choice of experimental animals for eye research. *Exp. Eye Res.*, 39:801–829, 1984.
20. Draize, J. H., Woodard, G., Calvery, H. L. Methods for the study of irritation and toxicity of substances applied topically to the skin and mucous membranes. *J. Pharmcol. Exp. Therap.*, 82:377–390, 1944.
21. Draize, J. H., Kelley, E. A. Toxicity to eye mucosa of certain cosmetic preparations containing surface-active agents. *Proc. Sci. Sect. Toilet Goods Assoc.*, 17:1–4, 1952.
22. Code of Federal Regulations Title 16, Part 1500.42. Washington, D.C., U.S. Government Printing Office, 1979.
23. Federal Hazard Substances Act Regulations, Code of Federal Regulations, 16, Part 1500, 1982.
24. Khodadoust, A. A., Green, K. Physiological function of regenerating epithelium. *Inves. Ophthalmol.*, 15:96–101, 1976.
25. Green, K. Corneal endothelial structure and function under normal and toxic conditions. *Curr. Biol. Revs.*, 25:169–207, 1981.

# *Chapter 4: Fibrin-Collagen Composite Tissue Adhesive*

D. H. SIERRA

## INTRODUCTION

Although they are the most successful surgical adhesives and sealants to date, fibrin sealants (FS) have a number of limitations in their mechanical and biological properties for certain applications. These limitations are more evident in the patient autologous or single-donor sourced FS preparations (derived from cryoprecipitation, ammonium sulfate precipitation, ethanol fractionation and other derivatives) than the commercially prepared pooled-source products, although they too share many of these shortcomings.

Among them are low viscosity prior to polymerization with thrombin, low cohesive strength after polymerization and short-term persistence ($<2$ weeks) in vivo. Low viscosity is problematic in microsurgical applications such as ossicular chain reconstruction in otologic surgery or peripheral nerve anastomosis. Low cohesive (mechanical) strength and short-term persistence due to proteolysis can lead to premature repair rupture in applications such as cerebrospinal fluid sealing in neurological repair or in vascular repair and anastomosis.

With these performance shortcomings in mind, coupled with the lack of a commercially available high-performance FS in the United States, a fibrin-collagen composite adhesive has been developed to overcome some of the physical limitations and consistency problems associated with the patient autologous and single-donor source FS products [1–3].

The fibrin-based composite tissue adhesive (CTA) composition is formulated by adding fibrillar type I collagen to fibrinogen-Factor XIII solutions to alter mechanical properties. This material could be used in place of FS or where FS is contraindicated because of inadequate mechanical performance.

The fibrinogen component can be obtained from a variety of sources and in almost any concentration. Upon the addition of low concentrations of thrombin, the flowable and moldable composite rapidly becomes a rigid adhesive mass.

A series of in vitro investigations to evaluate the effects of the addition of collagen to fibrin-sealant systems were performed. Collagen formulation, format and concentration effects upon gelation (thrombin) time was investigated. Prepolymerization viscosity and polymerized viscoelastic mechanical properties were also evaluated. In vitro and in vivo investigations into skin graft attachment [2], chemotherapeutic delivery [4], and cerebrospinal fluid leakage control [5] are described elsewhere. Clinical uses of the CTA are described in another chapter [6].

## MATERIALS AND METHODS

### Effect of Collagen Preparation on Gelation (Thrombin) Time

Experiments were performed to evaluate the effect of collagen preparation and buffer conditions on gelation times of purified bovine fibrinogen solutions (Sigma Chemical Co., St. Louis, MO). A total of 1 mL test solution was prepared and incubated at 37°C. To this, 10 $\mu$L of thrombin solution with $CaCl_2$ was added and mixed. The time for gelation or solidification was recorded. The test concentrations were:

[collagen]: 15–20 mg/mL
[fibrinogen]: 1.5 mg/mL
[thrombin]: 1 U/mL
[$Ca^{2+}$]: 20 mM
buffer pH: 7.2

The results are described in Table 4.1.

All test preparations were flowable, moldable viscoelastic fluids capable of being extruded through syringe hubs and/or needles prior to the addition of thrombin.

From the data, we conclude that for gelation enhancement to take place (gel time $< 5$ seconds)—the collagen would appear to be defined by a relatively narrow set of specifications—the collagen preparation must contain some significant percentage of fibers that are insoluble in the pH ranges useful for treatment in physiological conditions ($>$pH 5) and have a fiber diameter of 5 $\mu$m or greater. The collagen must be native (containing telopeptide ends) or near-native (lacking telopeptides). Treatments other

***Table 4.1.*** *Effect of collagen preparation and buffer condition on gelation times.*

| Sample ID # | Buffer (mM) [$Na^+$] | [$Cl^-$] | [$PO_4^{3-}$] | Collagen: Preparation Method (ref. #) | Other Treatments | Source | Telopeptides | Fiber Diameter $>5\ \mu m$ | Net Charge @ pH 7.2 | Gel Time (seconds) |
|---|---|---|---|---|---|---|---|---|---|---|
| 1 | 150 | 130 | 20 | 7 | none | corium | no | yes | physiologic | $<5$ |
| 2 | 150 | 130 | 20 | 7 | GTA x-linked | corium | no | yes | physiologic | $<5$ |
| 3 | 150 | 130 | 20 | 8 | none | corium | no | no | physiologic | $>300$ |
| 4 | 150 | 130 | 20 | 8 | incubated at 37°C for >2 h | corium | no | yes | physiologic | $<5$ |
| 5 | 236 | 68 | 100 | 8 | hypertonic | corium | no | no | physiologic | $>300$ |
| 6 | 236 | 68 | 100 | 8 | incubated at 37°C for >2 h | corium | no | yes | physiologic | $>300$ |
| 7 | 150 | 130 | 20 | [a] | none | tendon | no | yes | physiologic | $<5$ |
| 8 | 150 | 130 | 20 | [a] | GTA | tendon | no | yes | physiologic | $<5$ |
| 9 | 150 | 130 | 20 | 9 | succinylated | corium | yes | no | negative | $>300$ |
| 10 | 150 | 130 | 20 | 9 | succinylated | tendon | no | yes | negative | $>300$ |
| 11 | 150 | 130 | 20 | 10,11 | ionized HCl salt | corium | yes | yes | ? | 30 |
| 12 | 150 | 130 | 20 | [a] | contains bone minerals | cancellous bone | yes | yes | physiologic | $<5$ |

[a]Process details not available.

h = Hours.

GTA = Glutaraldehyde.

than cross-linking, such as succinylation [9] or ionization processing [10,11], would appear to inhibit gelation enhancement. The solvent conditions dictate physiologic or near physiologic pH and ionic strength. The formulations will gel under nonphysiologic conditions, however, at much slower rates.

### Concentrations and Gelation Time Effects in Vitro

The effects of collagen concentration upon gelation time of dilute fibrinogen preparations were investigated. The same assay conditions as those described in the previous study were used. Bovine fibrinogen was used for the dilute fibrinogen investigations (Sigma Chemical Co., St. Louis, MO).

The results for the dilute fibrinogen-collagen study are described in Figure 4.1.

As demonstrated using fibrinogen without collagen, there was some clotting effect at 0.07 and 0.035 mg/mL fibrinogen concentration. However, due to the fragility and fluidity of the resultant clots and comparison to the viscosity of a collagen-alone control using 6 mg/mL collagen, it was difficult to discern any clotting effect at these lower fibrinogen concentrations. As shown in Table 4.2, solid clots were achieved at fibrinogen concentrations of from 2.5 to 0.15 mg/mL using 6 mg/mL collagen.

This data demonstrated the practical limits for concentrations that can be used under these experimental conditions for dilute fibrinogen. In particular, compositions with concentrations of fibrinogen as high as 2.5 mg/mL gelled instantly and were not useful. Concentrations of 0.07 mg/mL or less produced a fluid and fragile clot. Formulations using between 1.25 and 0.15 mg/mL fibrinogen together with 15 mg/mL collagen produced useful adhesive compositions. Higher concentrations than 20 mg/mL of collagen may be used successfully.

Gelation of CTA formulations with fibrillar-collagen concentrations greater than 20 mg/mL is difficult to determine due to the high viscosity of the test solution. The highest concentration was at 32 mg/mL in both plasma and purified bovine fibrinogen (1.5 mg/mL fibrinogen concentration for both) under standard test conditions. The gelation times were 8 seconds and $<1$ second, respectively. Samples have been successfully produced with collagen concentrations as high as 60 mg/mL with as little as 1.5 mg/mL fibrin concentration. Higher collagen concentrations could be used with higher fibrinogen concentrations.

Higher concentrations of fibrinogen in the form of cryoprecipitate and with commercially prepared FS (Tissucol®) have also demonstrated accelerated gelation times. Fibrinogen concentrations up to 20 mg/mL have

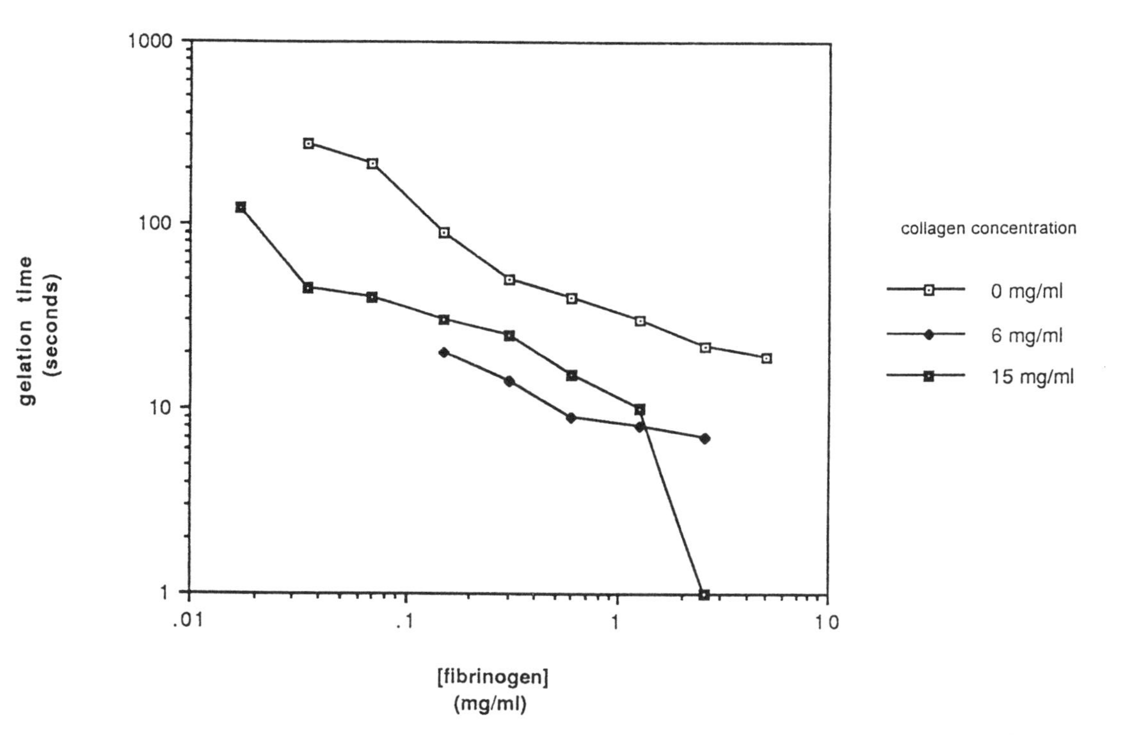


**FIGURE 4.1**
In vitro gelation (thrombin) time.

*Table 4.2. Gelation (thrombin) time.*

| Fibrinogen (mg/mL) | Collagen (mg/mL): | Gelation Time (seconds) | | |
|---|---|---|---|---|
| | | 0 | 6 | 15 |
| 5.000 | | 19 | <5 | <5 |
| 2.5 | | 22 | 7 | <5 |
| 1.25 | | 30 | 8 | 10 |
| 0.6 | | 40 | 9 | 15 |
| 0.3 | | 50 | 14 | 25 |
| 0.15 | | 90 | 20 | 30 |
| 0.07 | | 210 | n.g. | 40 |
| 0.035 | | 270 | n.g. | 45 |
| 0.017 | | n.g. | n.g. | 120 |
| 0.008 | | n.g. | n.g. | n.g. |

n.g.: No gelation noted.

demonstrated instantaneous gelation times with collagen concentrations up to 30 mg/mL. However, thrombin concentrations of 10 U/mL are required. Fibrinogen-only controls at these concentrations demonstrated gelation times of thirty seconds (unpublished results). Concentrations above these are difficult to evaluate due to the high viscosity of the preparations.

## Viscosity of Fibrinogen, Collagen and Composite Solutions; Prepolymerized

Studies were performed to evaluate the viscosity characteristics of fibrinogen, collagen, and CTA formulations prior to the addition of thrombin. The purpose of these studies was to investigate the interaction of collagen with fibrinogen prior to polymerization. This is an important parameter to evaluate as flow characteristics will dictate the ease of delivery as well as cohesiveness of a bolus of the material once delivered to a repair site and prior to the addition of thrombin. Preparations of low viscosity will be more likely to migrate from the repair site as well as be less amenable to further molding and shaping.

Samples were prepared and evaluated on a Brookfield cone and plate viscometer with data analysis software on a personal computer. The test conditions were:

temperature: 20°C ($\pm$0.2°C)
$\omega$ range: 0.8 to 225 $s^{-1}$
$\omega$ reported: 8.2 $s^{-1}$
[$Na^+$]: 150 mM

[$Cl^-$]: 130 mM
[$PO_4 3-$]: 20 mM
pH: 7.2

The results are described in Table 4.3.

The fibrinogen preparations with increasing fibrinogen concentration demonstrated an increase in viscosity and shear stress. The fibrillar collagen had a much higher viscosity and shear stress than the FS preparations. Upon mixing the fibrillar collagen with the cryoprecipitate and purified fibrinogen (results not reported here), the viscosity and shear rates undergo an unexpected increase greater than the expected additive increase in viscosity (appr. 2900 calculated vs 3662 cps) and shear stress (appr. 145 vs 302 dyne/$cm^2$). The CTA formulation incorporating plasma has an even higher viscosity than the collagen cryoprecipitate or concentrate version.

## Viscoelastic Mechanical Properties

The shear (torsional) viscoelastic mechanical properties of polymerized CTA and FS (cryoprecipitate) were characterized by molding specimens of different formulations into discs and evaluated on a thermostated parallel plate apparatus (Rheometrics Fluid Spectrometer). The test conditions were:

percent strain: 1%
strain rate: 0.1 to 800 $s^{-1}$
temperature: 24°C
[thrombin]: 1 U/mL
[$\epsilon$-aminocaproic acid]: 20 mg/mL (added as an antifibrinolytic for specimen stability)
[$Ca^{2+}$]: 20 mM
incubation time: 24 h before testing

***Table 4.3.*** *Viscosity of fibrinogen, collagen, and composite mixtures.*

| Sample ID # | Fibrinogen Source | Fibrinogen (mg/mL) | Collagen (mg/mL) | $\eta$ | $F$ |
|---|---|---|---|---|---|
| 1 | cryoprecipitate | 45 | 0 | 47.6 | 3.9 |
| 2 | purified | 120 | 0 | 142.7 | 11.8 |
| 3 | none | 0 | 32 | 1950 | 160.9 |
| 4 | cryoprecipitate | 22.5 | 32 | 3662 | 302.1 |
| 5 | plasma | 1.5 | 32 | 4423 | 364.9 |

$\eta$: Viscosity in centipoise (cps).
$F$: Shear stress in dyne/$cm^2$.

***Table 4.4.*** *Test formulations used in viscoelasticity study.*

| Sample ID # | Fibrin (mg/mL) | Collagen (mg/mL) | Total Protein (mg/mL) |
|---|---|---|---|
| 1 | 1.5 | 18 | 19.5 |
| 2 | 15 | 18 | 33 |
| 3 | 15 | 0 | 15 |

The sample formulations are described in Table 4.4 and the viscoelasticity results in Table 4.5.

The CTA formulations demonstrated higher storage modulus, loss modulus, and complex viscosity than FS formulations. The CTA samples also were found to have lower tan $\delta$ than FS at 30 mg/mL. CTA sample 2 demonstrated a higher complex modulus than the higher concentration FS as well as a lower loss over strain range.

The inclusion of collagen fibers significantly alters the mechanical properties of fibrin materials. Both the CTA formulations exhibited increases in storage, loss, and complex moduli and a decrease in tan $\delta$ when compared to FS. This is indicative of high binding strength between the collagen and fibrin. The CTA can thus be described as being "tougher"

***Table 4.5.*** *Viscoelastic properties of cryoprecipitate and CTA.*

| Sample #: | | 1 | 2 | 3 | 4 |
|---|---|---|---|---|---|
| $G'$ | 0.1 $s^{-1}$ | 6.2 | 20 | 2 | 5.5 |
| | 800 $s^{-1}$ | 17 | 33 | 5 | 15 |
| $G''$ | 0.1 $s^{-1}$ | 2 | 3.7 | 0.17 | 1.6 |
| | 800 $s^{-1}$ | 3 | 8 | 0.8 | 4 |
| $\eta^*$ | 0.1 $s^{-1}$ | 25 | 44 | 15 | 24 |
| | 800 $s^{-1}$ | 0.5 | 0.75 | 0.25 | 0.2 |
| tan $\delta$ | 0.1 $s^{-1}$ | 0.18 | 0.08 | – | 0.24 |
| | 800 $s^{-1}$ | 0.18 | 0.28 | – | 0.39 |
| | $\omega c$: | – | 250 | – | 5 |
| $G^*$ | 0%: | – | 25 | – | 13 |
| | 100% | – | 12 | – | 0.3 |

$G'$: Storage modulus.
$G''$: Loss modulus.
$\eta^*$: Complex viscosity.
tan $\delta$: $G''/G'$.
$G^*$: Complex modulus.
All values are (dyne/cm$^2$) × $10^2$ unless noted.

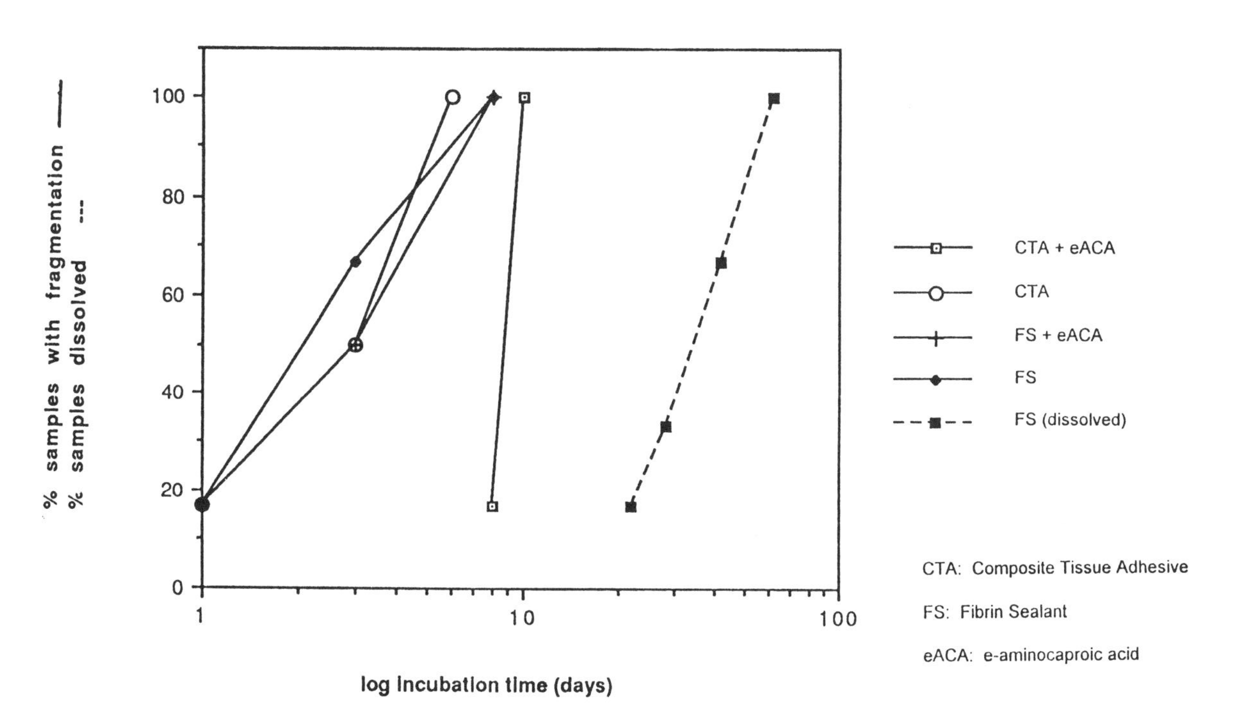


**FIGURE 4.2**
In vitro dissolution onset time.

than conventional FS based on protein content comparison. The improvement in mechanical strength could permit the use of CTA in clinical situations where FS would likely fail under mechanical stress, such as packing and sealing cerebrospinal fluid leakages in transdural procedures or securing arterial/venous access devices.

### Dissolution Onset Time

The time for onset of clot dissolution of CTA and FS formulations with and without the inclusion of an antifibrinolytic ($\epsilon$-aminocaproic acid) was investigated using a previously described method [12]. Cryoprecipitate was used as FS at a concentration of 20 mg/mL. Fibrillar collagen as described above was used at the same concentration. Thrombin concentration was 100 U/mL (Sigma Chemical Co., St. Louis, MO). The percentage of samples first exhibiting visible signs of degradation were recorded as a function of time. The results are described in Figure 4.2.

The addition of collagen or antifibrinolytic to FS did not appreciably decrease the onset of degradation. However, the addition of both collagen and antifibrinolytic significantly decreased the onset of degradation in a synergistic manner.

## CONCLUSION

The addition of type I fibrillar atelopeptide collagen appears to alter effectively the mechanical properties of FS regardless of the source or formulation. It appears from these studies and others that the biological and biochemical properties are altered as well. Further studies are required to understand the interaction between the components. The in vitro and in vivo wound healing characteristics still need to be evaluated in depth, thus defining the collagen-fibrinogen interaction and contributions to the performance of composite.

The ability to alter these parameters in FS allows greater flexibility in utilizing sealants and adhesives in situations where FS may not be useful or too limited. This is especially true of the single-donor and patient autologous preparations. As these parameters may be altered by adjusting the component concentrations, the adhesive formulation may be tailored for a specific application. For example, a high-fibrinogen, low-collagen concentration material could be used in skin graft attachment; it would possess low viscosity for rapid and thorough spreading over the graft bed, demonstrating high adhesive strength and sufficient flexibility to allow some motion without bond rupture. A lower-fibrinogen, high-collagen formulation could be used in either packing hard tissues or used as a "putty" with donor bone powder in craniofacial procedures or mastoid bone repair in mastoidectomies. High viscosity would greatly facilitate molding and maintaining shape prior to polymerization by allowing the surgeon ample time to attain the desired contouring. The high modulus attained after polymerization would minimize deformation during the healing process.

It is foreseeable that several different formulations of fibrin-based adhesives, with and without collagen, would be available to the surgeon, each with characteristics suitable for specific tissues, procedures or techniques. Thus, the best material for the job would be used, with little or no compromise in performance.

## REFERENCES

1. Sierra, D. H., Luck, E. E., Brown, D. M., Shieh, P. In vitro physico-chemical characteristics of a fibrin-based composite tissue adhesive. *Fourth World Biomater. Congr.* #366, 1992.
2. Sierra, D. H., Saltz, R., Price, M., Stowers, R., Luck, E. E., Brown, D. M. In vivo performance of a fibrin-based composite tissue adhesive. *Fourth World Biomat. Congr.* #367, 1992.
3. Sierra, D. H., Luck, E. E., Brown, D. M. Surgical adhesive material. U.S. patent 5,290,552, 1994.
4. Sierra, D. H., Luck, E. E., Brown, D. M. Yu, N. Y. Fibrin-collagen adhesive drug delivery system for tumor therapy. *Trans. Soc. Biomater.*, 16:257, 1993.
5. Sierra, D. H., Rock, J. P., Castro-Moure, F., Jiang, F., Kloss, J. M. Skullbase cerebrospinal fluid leakage control with a fibrin composite tissue adhesive. *Trans. Soc. Biomater.*, 20:245, 1995.
6. Sierra, D. H., Perkins, R. C. Clinical use of fibrin-based composite tissue adhesive in otology and neurotology. *Surgical Adhesives and Sealants: Current Technology and Applications*, D. H. Sierra, R. Saltz, eds. Technomic Publishing Co., Inc., Lancaster, PA, 1996.
7. Luck, E. E., Daniels, J. R. Non-antigenic collagen and articles of manufacture. U.S. patent 4,233,360, 1978.
8. Daniels, J. R., Knapp, T. R. Process for augmenting connective mammalian tissue with in situ polymerizable native collagen solution. U.S. patent 3,949,0773, 1976.
9. Miyata, T., Rubin, A. L., Stenzel, K. H., Dunn, M. W. Collagen drug delivery device. U.S. patent 4,164,559, 1979.
10. Battista, O. A. Microcrystalline collagen, an ionizable partial salt of collagen and foods, pharmaceuticals and cosmetics containing the same. U.S. Patent 3,628,974, 1973.
11. Battista, O. A., Cruz, M. M., Hait, M. R. Fibrous collagen derived product having hemostatic and wound binding properties. U.S. patent 3,742,955, 1973.
12. Harris, D. H., Siedentop, K. H., Ham, K. R., Sanchez, B. Autologous fibrin tissue adhesive biodegradation and systemic effects. *Laryngoscope*, 97:1141 – 1144, 1987.

# *Chapter 5: Soldering Is a Superior Alternative to Fibrin Sealant*

L. S. BASS, S. K. LIBUTTI, M. L. KAYTON,
R. NOWYGROD and M. R. TREAT

## INTRODUCTION

Fibrin sealant has been quite useful for hemostasis in many surgical applications [1]. Attempts to use this process for tissue bonding are only partly successful. Advantages include elimination of tissue trauma and foreign body response of sutures, speed, and ease. Unlike suture repairs, adhesive repairs tend to be immediately watertight, which is particularly useful for vascular, gastrointestinal, and urologic applications. Experimental studies of skin closure [2], bronchial stump leakage [3], and nerve repair [4] have shown some success. Immediate tensile strength has been marginal and limitations include short shelf life, variable handling characteristics, and risk of blood-borne pathogens, such as hepatitis and HIV. Recent advances have allowed virus inactivation using a solvent/detergent treatment, reducing the risk of disease transmission [5]. At the time of this writing, no FDA-approved commercial product is available in the United States, but individual blood-bank products are formulated at some hospitals for clinicians. In addition, several products have been used for over a decade in Europe (e.g., Tissucol®).

Laser welding is another technique that has been studied in multiple systems. While immediate weld strength is superior to that obtained with fibrin glue, it remains marginal. Despite the possibility of reduced scarring and stenosis, significant thermal injury is created producing other complications, such as aneurysms [6,7]. Stay sutures are often required for strength and coaptation.

A modification of this technique, termed "laser soldering," involves the addition of substrate to the weld site to increase weld strength. By application of a proteinaceous material to the weld site prior to laser welding, several advantages accrue [8,9]. Weld strength is increased while thermal injury is decreased. Coaptations are also reduced. Despite these advantages, solder performance has been highly variable. Fibrin adhesive and staple closure were compared to laser soldering with cryoprecipitate and with a new laser solder for closure of skin incisions in the rat model.

## MATERIALS AND METHODS

### Laser System

A portable, air-cooled, gallium-aluminum-arsenide diode laser (Surgimedics Inc., The Woodlands, TX) was used with a 400 $\mu$m core diameter flexible quartz fiber. The laser had an output wavelength of 810 nm. Power output was 3 W, spot size 2 mm, power density 95.5 W/cm$^2$.

### Preparation of Adhesives/Solders

Cryoprecipitate was derived from pooled human plasma that had been subjected to solvent/detergent treatment (The New York Blood Center, New York, NY) [5]. Cryoprecipitate had a total protein concentration of 79.4 $\pm$7.6 mg/mL and a fibrinogen concentration of 9.9 $\pm$0.9 mg/mL. Tubes containing 3 mL cryoprecipitate were stored at $-80$°C. Immediately before use, each tube was warmed to 37°C. The final preparation was an easily-derived, viscous fluid that was turbid. For laser activation, tubes were mixed with 1.5 mg of indocyanine green dye (ICG) (Becton-Dickinson, Cockeysville, MD). Bovine thrombin (Thrombostat, Parke-Davis, Morris Plains, NJ) was mixed in Tris buffer to a concentration of 20 U/mL with 20 mM calcium chloride. Thrombin was stored at $-80$°C and thawed immediately prior to use. Cryoprecipitate and thrombin were applied to wounds simultaneously through a double-barrelled syringe, allowing precise 1:1 mixing during application.

Laser solder was prepared as a mixture of human albumin (The New York Blood Center, Melville Biologics Division, New York, NY), sodium hyaluronate (Healon™ Kabi Pharmacial Ophthalmics, Inc., Monrovia, CA) and ICG. Final concentrations were: albumin 18.5%, hyaluronate 0.5%, ICG 0.05%. ICG has a peak absorption at 805 nm, closely matched to the laser wavelength selected.

Soldering was performed by applying a thin layer of the solder material to the apposed skin edges. The solder was then exposed to laser light until lightening and shrinkage were maximal but before any charring or desiccation were produced. This represented the end point of welding.

### Animal Model

Male Sprague-Dawley rats were anesthetized with ketamine and xylazine. The back of each animal was shaved and painted with povidone-iodine solution. Longitudinal skin incisions three centimeters in length were made on the dorsum. Two surgical staples were placed at the extreme ends of each incision to gently appose the wound edges. Incisions were then closed with one of four techniques: (1) staples; (2) thrombin-activated cryoprecipitate (fibrin sealant); (3) laser-activated cryoprecipitate; (4) laser-activated multicomponent solder. Control rats were closed with three additional surgical skin staples. Specimens were harvested for analysis at time periods ranging from zero hours to four days.

### Analysis

Skin staples were removed prior to tensile strength determination. Skin strips were harvested and cross sectional areas measured with calipers. Strips were then mounted on a T10 Tensiometer (Monsanto, Akron, OH), with a crosshead speed of 10 mm/min., for determination of peak breaking strength. Individual tensile strength determinations were averaged to arrive at a mean value for each animal. Mean tensile strengths between techniques and timepoints were compared by ANOVA. Additional skin segments were harvested and fixed in 10% buffered formalin for histologic analysis. After paraffin embedding and sectioning, specimens were stained with hematoxylin and eosin. Samples were evaluated for thermal damage and inflammation.

## RESULTS

Tensile strength values are expressed in Table 5.1. At all timepoints, laser-activated solders were significantly stronger than thrombin-activated cryoprecipitate ($p < 0.01$) and control wounds ($p < 0.003$). Eight samples were tested in each group. There was no significant difference in tensile strength between the two laser solders at any timepoint. At time zero, solder closures had mean strengths comparable to a stapled closure at four days.

Gross examination showed no charring in either laser group. Thermal injury was confined to the solder and superficial layers of the dermis. Solder engendered no inflammation in comparison with control specimens.

***Table 5.1.*** *Mean tensile strength (g/cm²).*

| Technique | Day 0 | Day 4 |
|---|---|---|
| Staples | – | 53 ± 77 |
| Fibrin Sealant | 99 ± 6 | 733 ? 35 |
| Cryoprecipitate-Laser | 570 ± 35 | 779 ± 64 |
| Multisolder-Laser | 482 ± 15 | 668 ± 101 |

## DISCUSSION

In this study, laser soldering produced superior weld strength compared with fibrin sealant. Cryoprecipitate is a suitable source of fibrinogen [10]. Soldered fibrinogen is probably denatured and does not proceed to fibrin formation. Oz et al. showed that urokinase was unable to weaken a cryoprecipitate laser-soldered vascular anastomosis [11]. Strength is only one of several relevant parameters. Cost, ease-of-application, or other biomechanical parameters such as elasticity, were not evaluated. Long-term follow-up on wounds may demonstrate later thermal effects on wound healing that were not apparent by four days.

Laser soldering proves superior when compared with laser welding [12]. Weld strength is greatly improved, thermal injury reduced, and coaptation simplified. Fibrin sealants, while an attractive alternative, do not offer comparable results and control for most applications. The task of preparing cryoprecipitate from autologous or banked blood can be cumbersome. The resulting product is limited in amount and shelf life. Its need must be anticipated preoperatively. Initial tensile strength is significantly lower than laser soldering. The effect is not instantaneous and the end point cannot be clearly judged by the surgeon. Laser soldering allows the surgeon to weld in many layers if desired and to a visually determined end point. Laser soldering may be less suited for flap fixation where the flap is too thick to be transilluminated by the laser light. For this application the large flap area can be quickly fixed by fibrin sealants. Routine use of soldering for simple hemostasis seems to be unnecessarily complex.

Laser soldering does add the cost and complexity of a laser. However, most clinically available lasers, as well as electrocautery units, are capable of performing soldering. A safe, effective weld is more easily created when using solder, reducing technical and judgement demands on the surgeon. Moreover, the solder represents a uniform target that can be expected to have a similar response every time despite variations in tissue. This allows rapid learning of the necessary end point by the surgeon.

While many lasers can be used for soldering, the technique described here is preferable [7]. Diode lasers are inexpensive, compact, and reliable with current indications for ophthalmic, urologic, and general surgical photocoagulation. The 810 nm wavelength lies at a similar optical range for nonpigmented body tissues. This means that at low power densities, there is little effect on unstained tissue. By mixing the ICG into the solder it is possible to create a photoenhancement effect that provides marked absorption of the laser light in the solder with little direct heating of native tissues. This allows the use of a lower-power, laser-reducing cost and less risk to the eye in the operating room. It also significantly reduces collateral thermal injury.

Laser soldering could play a significant role in surgical hemostasis, sealing of leaky anastomoses (e.g., vascular, biliary, urologic), and for tissue bonding. Tissue-bonding areas where laser soldering could offer potential advantages over suture techniques include microsurgery, graft fixation, laparoscopic surgery, and anastomoses that must be watertight. The solder could also act as a drug-delivery vehicle for growth factors, antibiotics, or a variety of other therapeutic agents.

A new laser solder has been developed with comparable strength to cryoprecipitate solder and additional advantages of improved handling properties, shelf life, sterility, and easy availability. Further study is needed to insure that these materials are fully biocompatible and retain strength during healing. The nature of the precursors, which are normally found in a healing wound, provide a theoretical basis for this to be acceptable. Laser soldering provides a powerful new technique for sealing, hemostasis, and tissue closure. The applications in which this provides a clinical advantage over conventional techniques must now be defined.

## REFERENCES

1. Matthew, T. L., Spotnitz, W. D., Kron, I. L., Daniel, T. M., Tribble, C. G., Nolan, S. P. Four years' experience with fibrin sealant in thoracic and cardiovascular surgery. *Ann. Thorac. Surg.*, 50:40–44, 1990.
2. Saltz, R., Sierra, D., Feldman, D., Saltz, M. B., Dimick, A., Vasconez, L. O. Experimental and clinical applications of fibrin glue. *Plast. Recontr. Surg.*, 88:104–114, 1991.
3. Glover, W., Chavis, T. V., Daniel, T. M., Kron, I. L., Spotnitz, W. D. Fibrin glue application through the flexible fiberoptic bronchoscope: Closure of bronchopleural fistulas. *J. Thorac. Cardiovas. Surg.*, 93:470–473, 1987.
4. Maragj, J., Meuer, B. S., Davenport, D., Gould, K. D., Terzis, J. K. Morphofunctional evaluation of fibrin glue versus microsuture nerve repairs. *J. Reconstr. Microsurg.*, 6:331–337, 1990.
5. Horowitz, B., Bonomo, R., Prince, A. M., Chin, S. N., Brotman, B., Shulman, R. W. Solvent/detergent-treated plasma: A virus-inactivated substitute for fresh plasma. *Blood,* 79:826–831, 1992.

6. McCarthy, W., LoCicero, J., Hartz, R. S., Yao, J. S. T. Patency of laser-assisted anastomoses in small vessels: One year follow-up. *Surgery,* 102:319–326, 1986.
7. Oz, M. C., Chuck, R. S., Johnson, J. P., Parangi, S., Bass, L. S., Nowygrod, R., Treat, M. R. Indocyanine green dye enhanced vascular welding with the near infrared diode laser. *Vasc. Surg.*, 24:564, 1990.
8. Poppas, D. P., Schlossberg, S. M., Richmond, I. L., Gilbert, D. A., Devine, C. J. Laser welding in urethral surgery: Improved results with a protein solder. *J. Urol.*, 139:415–417, 1988.
9. Grubbs, P. E., Marini, C. C., Basu, S., Rose, D. M., Cunningham, J. N. Enhancement of $CO_2$ laser microvascular anastomoses fibrin glue. *J. Surg. Res.*, 45:112–119, 1988.
10. Marx, G., Blankenfield, A. Kinetic and mechanical parameters of pure and cryoprecipitate fibrin. *Blood Coag. Fibrin,* 4:73–78, 1992.
11. Oz, M. C., Bass, L. S., Chuck, R. S., Johnson, J. P., Prangi, S., Nowygrod, R., Treat, M. R. Strength of laser vascular fusion: Preliminary observations on the role of thrombus. *Laser Surg. Med.*, 10:393–395, 1990.
12. Oz, M. C., Johnson, J. P., Parangi, S., Chuck, R. S., Marboe, C. C. Bass, L. S., Nowygrod, R., Treat, M. R. Tissue soldering by use of indocyanine green dye-enhanced fibrinogen with the near infrared diode laser. *J. Vasc. Surg.*, 11:718–725, 1990.

# SECTION II

# LABORATORY EVALUATION

# *Chapter 6: Kinetic and Mechanical Parameters of Fibrin Glue*

G. MARX

## INTRODUCTION

Fibrin glue (FG) is the quintessential, albeit concentrated version of fibrin formed as a result of physiological blood coagulation. FG is prepared in a two-component form as fibrinogen and thrombin. Its potential as a clinical tool makes it worth characterizing in some detail the mechanism of its formation as well as FG biochemical and biophysical properties. This chapter describes some general factors of FG formation and its properties, particularly as they are modulated by the universal parameters of ionic strength ($\mu$) and pH.

## MECHANISM OF GEL FORMATION

The transformation of soluble fibrinogen into fibrin gel involves enzymatic as well as polymerization reactions (review in References [1−6]). Two distinct polymerization steps contribute to gelation. Initially, thrombin activate fibrinogen by enzymatically cleaving fibrinopeptide A (FPA). The resultant monomers are unstable and spontaneously form linear multimers (or oligomers) called "protofibrils." The activation of fibrinogen by thrombin (or another enzyme such as reptilase) generates monomeric units of fibrin that elongate the protofibrils. These eventually react with one another by lateral association, which results in branching and the formation of a three-dimensional gel network. The latter step is accelerated by divalent cations, notably physiologic levels of Ca(II) and Zn(II) [4,5]. Another means by which branching and network formation can occur is by occasional trinodular junction formation within the protofibril chain [6]. These reactions are responsible for

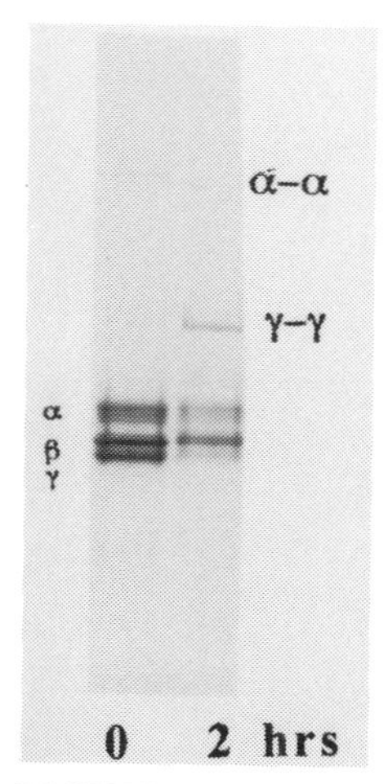


**FIGURE 6.1**
Reduced SDS-PAGE of FG at times 0 and 2 hours after mixing the fibrinogen with thrombin components. The loss of $\alpha$ and $\gamma$ band can be seen and the rise of $\gamma$-$\gamma$ dimers as well as $(\alpha\text{-}\alpha)_n$ multimers can be seen. These covalent multimers are due to Factor XIIIa-induced crosslinking of fibrin fibers.

the formation of the nucleating gel structure, which is detected by monitoring clotting time (CT).

After the onset of gelation, further units of fibrin are deposited onto the nucleating gel, and the resulting network becomes thicker and denser. Factor XIII, which is usually present in fibrinogen preparations, is also activated by thrombin to form an active transglutaminase (Factor XIIIa) which covalently cross links $\alpha$ and $\gamma$ chains of different fibrin monomers in the gel [7,9]. This is illustrated in Figure 6.1 that presents a typical reduced electrophoretic gel of FG at zero and two hours after mixing the components. It shows the loss of the $\alpha$ and $\gamma$ chains of the fibrinogen and the rise of $\alpha$-$\alpha$ multimers and $\gamma$-$\gamma$ dimers. The cross-links can be ascribed to the Ca(II)-dependent XIIIa reactions. Factor XIIIa also covalently anchors the fibrin to cellular receptors and tissue sites. In many cases, these cross-links greatly increase the mechanical properties of the resultant fibrin as will be discussed later.

## KINETICS OF GELATION

The rate at which fibrin gel forms (expressed at clotting time, CT) is dependent on both the thrombin and fibrinogen levels, though their rate dependencies vary in a complex manner. For example, the rate of gelation

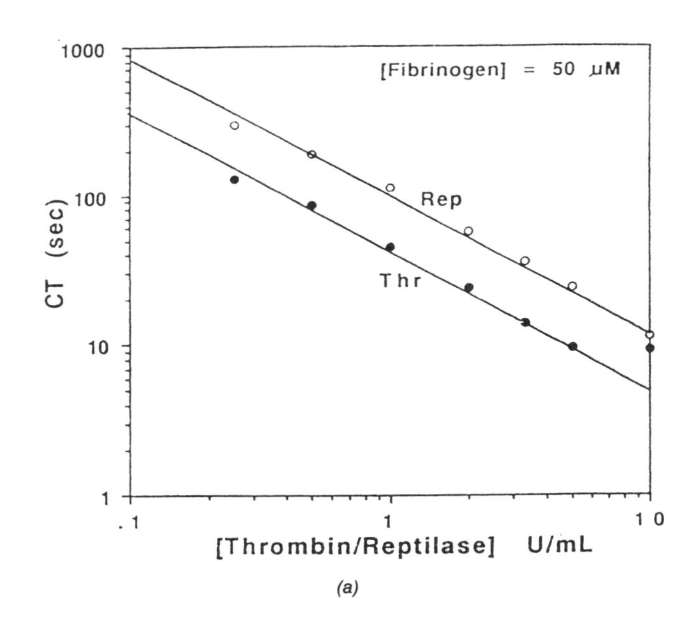


(a)

Fibrin Clotting Time

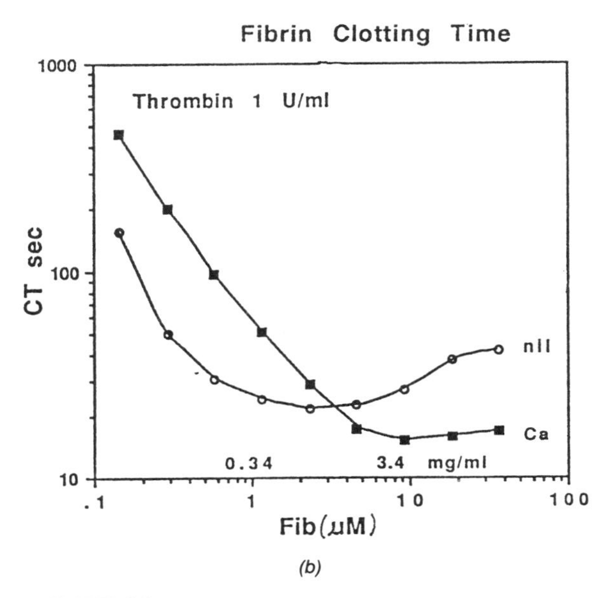


(b)

**FIGURE 6.2**
(a) Clotting time (CT) of 2 mg/mL pure fibrinogen induced by various levels of thrombin or reptilase. A decrease in CT reflects an increased rate of gelation. (b) Thrombin-induced (1 U/mL) CT at different concentrations of fibrinogen, without and with 2.5 mM Ca(II). The biphasic dependency of the CT on fibrinogen levels makes it difficult to predict CT.

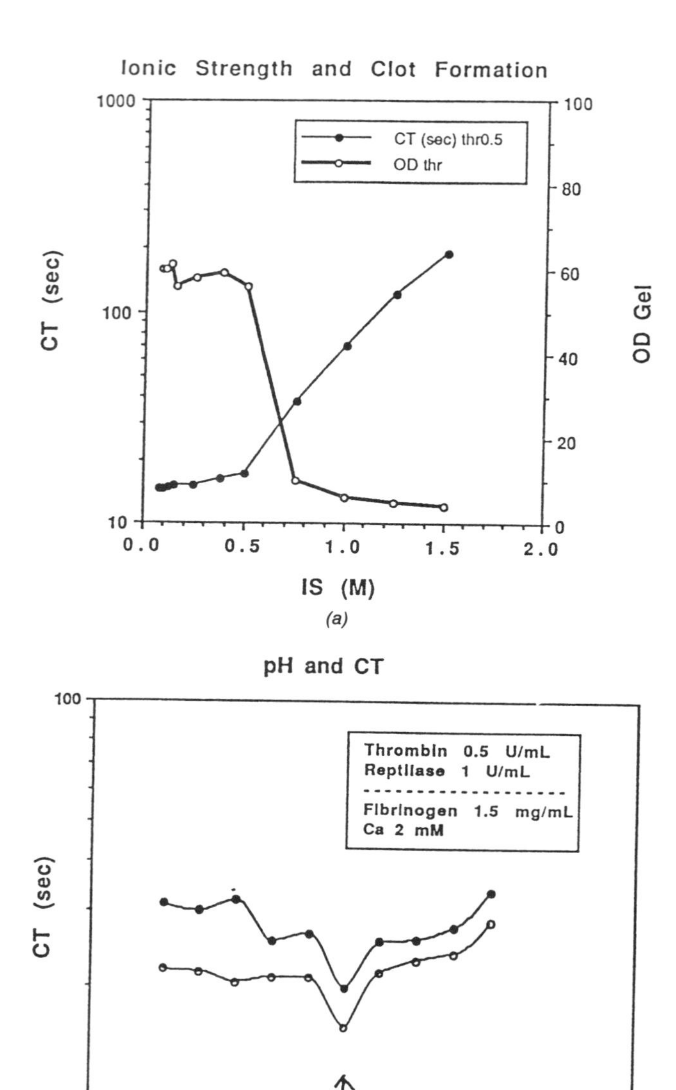


**FIGURE 6.3**
(a) Effect of ionic strength (IS) on clotting time (CT). It seems that the CT is not overly sensitive to IS except when it exceeds 0.5 M. These data show that CT is near optimum near physiologic IS of 0.15 M. For contrast, the turbidity (as $ABS_{600nm}$) of the same fibrin is presented. Higher turbidity reflects thicker fibrin fibers. (b) CT of thrombin- or reptilase-induced fibrin with 2 mM Ca(II) as affected by pH. The minimum value achieved at pH 7.4 shows that fibrin is formed most rapidly at physiologic pH.

(log CT) is inversely proportional to thrombin (or reptilase) levels at a fixed level of pure fibrinogen [Figure 6.2(a)]. One should be aware that below ten seconds, limitations of the instrumentation and mechanical handling prevent quantitation of CT so that these are effectively instantaneous.

By contrast, the CT exhibits biphasic dependency on fibrinogen levels at a fixed level of thrombin [Figure 6.2(b)]. Outside the range of 1 – 10 mg/mL fibrinogen, the CT increases either with increased or with decreased fibrinogen levels. This indicates that two distinct processes are impacting the rate of gelation.

Simulation kinetic models developed in this laboratory suggest that these complex kinetics may be due to the binding of protofibrils with unreacted fibrinogen. That is, protofibrils can form complexes with starting fibrinogen. The formation of fibrinogen:protofibril complexes has been amply demonstrated [10 – 13]. Such complexes are less capable of lateral polymerization associations. In FG, which usually contains high levels of fibrinogen ($>$ 10 mg/mL), intermediate fibrinogen:protofibril inhibit lateral association reactions, which results in a decreased rate of coagulation (increased CT).

The multitude of operative mechanisms prevents a simple calculation of CT for a particular FG formulation. In practice, one needs to carry out a small-scale test on the FG of choice to determine the CT of a particular combination of thrombin and fibrinogen.

Two universal physical chemical parameters that influence the rate of fibrin gel formation include ionic strength (IS, or, $\mu$) and pH. Because of their importance, data relating to their effects on CT are presented here. For example, relatively low IS that encompasses the physiologic value of 0.15 N can be seen to have only a minor effect on CT [Figure 6.3(a)], though CT increases almost linearly above 0.5 M. This is interesting from the point of view of fabricating FG devices in vitro, but has little impact on FG applied topically that is formulated at physiologic $\mu$.

The effect of pH on CT is rather different. It was observed that the physiologic level (pH 7.4) is actually the one at which coagulation is most rapid (lowest CT) [Figure 6.3(b)]. The coagulation rate of thrombin or reptilase-induced fibrin is slower above or below the optimum value pH 7.4. These data indicate that FG coagulation is most rapid at physiologic conditions.

## MECHANICAL PROPERTIES

### Viscoelasticity

Viscoelasticity is a difficult parameter to evaluate and to describe [14]. It relates to the ability of a material to remain flexible and to retain its shape, even after it has been deformed, for example, as by stretching or bending. Clearly, viscoelasticity is important in a biological adhesive that is to be applied to a flexible system, such as soft tissue. This is a major distinction of adhesives that are applied to structurally static systems, such as teeth or bones.

Nevertheless, little work has been done on the viscoelasticity of FG, though one can refer to work carried out at low fibrinogen-level fibrin [(Reference [15] and references therein)]. Part of this is due to limitations of the instrumentation. For example, the thromboelastograph used in some coagulation laboratories that measures the complex modulus ($G^*$), has a very low dynamic range. That is, the amplitude of the instrument is easily achieved with 10 mg/mL fibrin. This makes it difficult to evaluate the $G^*$ of more concentrated formulations of FG.

Nonetheless, because it shows the "real time" development of an important physical property during fibrin maturation and cross-linking, it is worth describing the viscoelastic behavior of fibrin in a few contexts. For example, the effect of Ca(II)-dependent cross-linking can be seen in the dynamic viscoelasticity development [Figure 6.4(a)]. Here, the effect of Ca(II) or its withdrawal (with EDTA) can be monitored in the real-time development of viscoelastic behavior. Cross-linking is clearly important in determining the final $G^*$ of the fibrin, and it requires somewhat longer to maximize than the initial onset of gelation, which here took less than one minute. Thus, we learn that the development of maximal viscoelastic properties of fibrin take much longer than would be expected from CT measurements.

Another experiment was designed to evaluate the effect of $\mu$ on the maximal viscoelasticity of fibrin. It was observed that the physiologic $\mu$ was the one at which maximal viscoelasticity was exhibited. These data conform to the data obtained on CT (see above) and point to physiologic conditions as the ones in which FG should be formulated. While these experiments show that viscoelasticity is useful, it is too difficult to measure in the range of interest (fibrinogen $>$ 10 mg/mL) for investigators examining or monitoring FG.

## Breaking Strength

Breaking strength (BS) of FG is of major interest because this reflects its utility in terms of one of its intended applications. BS is distinct from adhesion to skin or other tissue in that it only reflects the internal interaction of fibrin. It does not reflect binding or cross-linking to cellular sites or to other materials; thus, BS is entirely self-referential.

BS is greatly affected by cross-linking induced by Factor XIII. By either removing Factor XIII, or by not adding Ca(II) or chelating it with EDTA,

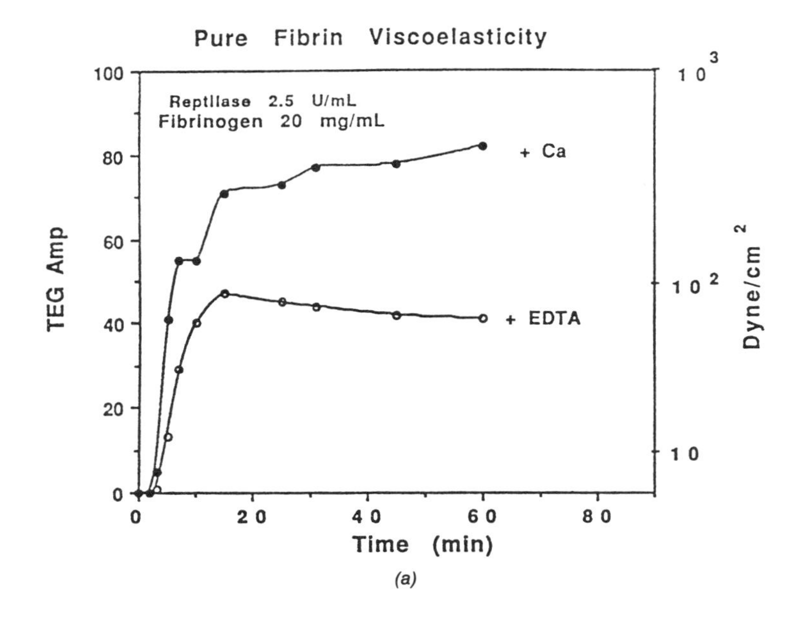


(a)

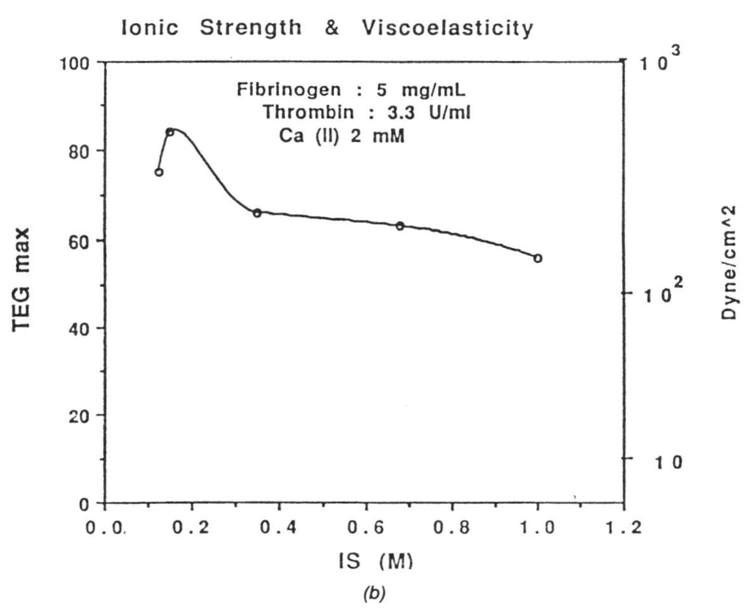


(b)

**FIGURE 6.4**
(a) Thromboelastograph viscoelastic development (as TEG amplitude) or reptilase-induced fibrin without or with Ca(II) or the chelator EDTA. Ca(II) clearly contributes to the rate of maximal viscoelasticity of the fibrin. (b) Maximum viscoelasticity ($TEG_{max}$) of fibrin after two hours incubation formed at various ionic strength (IS). The peak at 0.15 M reflects the viscoelasticity of fibrin under physiologic $\mu$.

one can estimate the contribution of cross-linking to the mechanical properties of FG. For example, a test was developed for measuring the BS by mixing FG components in a plastic test tube and pipetting the still-liquid mixture into the interface of two pieces of coarse, synthetic mesh (0.4 cm thick × 1 cm wide), allowing the formation of gel totally interwoven between the two pieces of coarse mesh [16]. After two hours, which allows the Factor XIIIa-induced cross-linking reaction [see viscoelasticity data Figure 6.4(a)], the mesh-fibrin-mesh ensemble was pulled apart and the BS was measured as grams per 0.4 $cm^2$ cross-section.

In such a test system, the BS of FG activated with thrombin without or with 2.5 mM Ca(II) exhibits a linear correlation fibrinogen concentration (Figure 6.5) as described by:

$$BS = slope * [Fib]$$

where [Fib] = fibrinogen concentration.

Over a range of fibrinogen levels, the slope of FG formed with Ca(II)

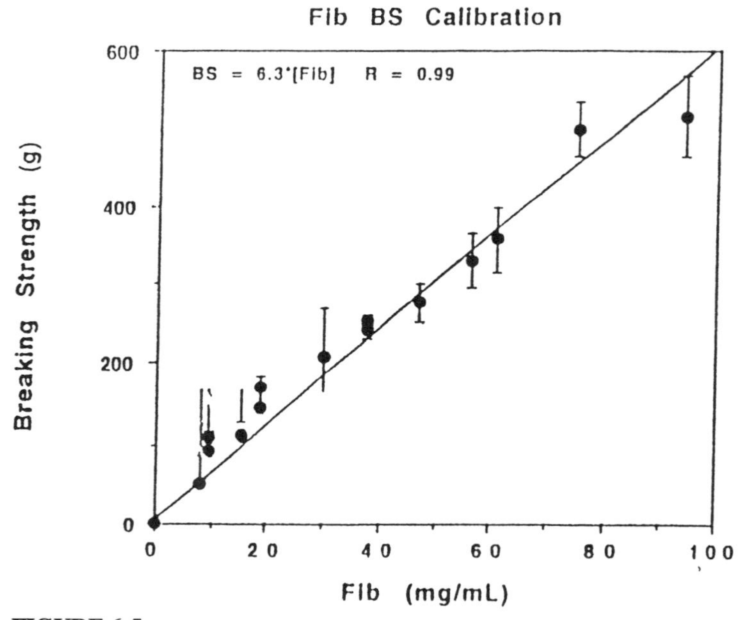


**FIGURE 6.5**
The BS (in g required to break a 0.4 $cm^2$ cross section) of FG at different fibrinogen levels with 5 U/mL thrombin and 10 mM Ca(II). The slope of this preparation gives a BS index of 6.3 g per mg/mL.

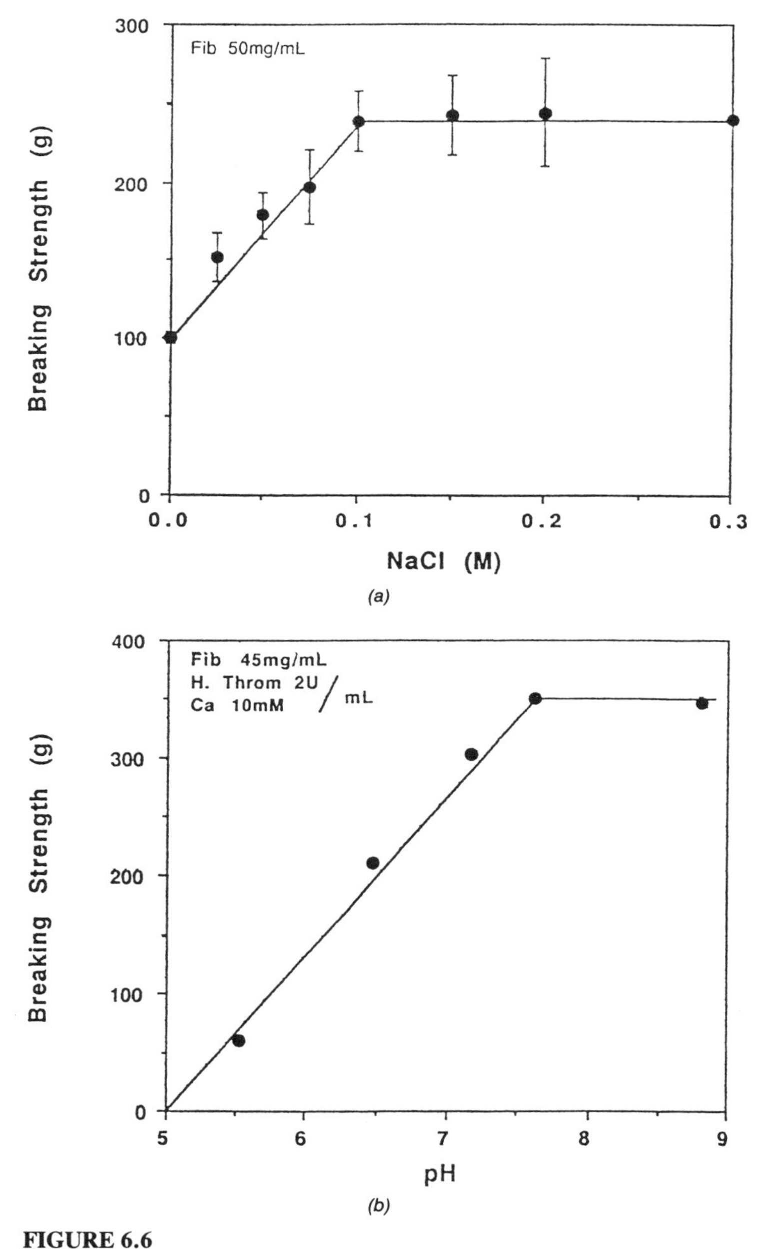


**FIGURE 6.6**
(a) Effect of varying ionic strength ($\mu$) on the BS of FG (at 50 mg/mL fibrinogen). The BS is low at low $\mu$ and plateaus above 0.1 M. (b) Effect of varying pH on the BS of FG (at 45 mg/mL fibrinogen). The BS is low at low pH but plateaus sharply at and above pH 7.4. This means that FG formulations will have optimum BS characteristics at physiologic pH.

was significantly larger than FG formed without Ca(II) (not shown). The higher slope reveals the contribution of Ca(II)-dependent Factor XIIIa-induced cross-linking. Actually, the slope of the BS versus fibrinogen levels is also helpful in evaluating the usefulness of FG preparation. That is, for a single fibrinogen level, one can measure the BS of a particular preparation or formulation. Dividing this by the fibrinogen level generates a number (BS index, with units of g per mg/mL) that reflects the innate strength of that FG preparation. The larger the value of the BS index, the stronger the FG preparation or formulation.

The effects of $\mu$ and pH on FG breaking strength were examined. BS plateaus at 0.1 N NaC1 [Figure 6.6(a)] were observed. This is well before the physiologic value of 0.15 N and shows the relative insensitivity of FG to $\mu$.

By contrast, the BS maximizes almost exactly at the physiologic pH of 7.4, and plateaus thereafter [Figure 6.6(b)]. The contrast between these experiments is revealing. In conjunction with the CT dependencies on $\mu$ and pH (Figure 6.3), it suggests that the molecular associations of monomers within the fibrin fibers are more severely dictated by hydrogen bonding than by charge-charge ionic interactions or by van der Waals forces.

## CONCLUSION

This study evaluates the effects of a few universal parameters such as concentration, $\mu$ and pH on the kinetics of formation and the physical properties of FG. The techniques described here are informative in that they demonstrate that FG in vitro is optimal at physiological conditions of pH and ionic strength. As viral sterilization methods will be applied to licensed FG, these techniques will help certify that the sterilizing techniques do not affect negatively the mechanical properties of the FG components. Similar evaluations should be made for additives to FG. Notwithstanding in vitro evaluations, biologic considerations dictate that FG be optimized with in vivo models. These studies suggest that the biologic/clinical potential of FG can be best achieved if it is developed with reference to its biochemistry and biophysics.

## ACKNOWLEDGEMENT

I wish to thank colleagues and associates who contributed to various aspects of this work including X. Mou, E. Sanchez, and R. Freed who work in my laboratory.

## REFERENCES

1. Hantgan R., McDonagh, J., Hermans, J. Fibrin assembly. *Ann. N.Y. Acad. Sci.*, 408:344–346, 1983.
2. Blomback, B. Fibrinogen and fibrin formation and its role in fibrinolysis. In: *Biotechnology of Blood.* Chapter 11. J. Goldstein, ed.
3. Kerenyi, G. Polymers of natural origin as biomaterial. I., Fibrin. *Macromolecular Biomaterials.* Chapter 4. B. W. Hastings, P. Ducheyne , eds. CRC Press, Boca Raton, Florida, 1984.
4. Marx G. Mechanism of fibrin coagulation based on selective, cation-driven, protofibril association. *Biopolymers,* 27:763–774, 1988.
5. Marx G. Modelling (proto) fibrin coagulation. *Biopolymers,* 29:1233–1241, 1990.
6. Mosesson, M., DiOrio, J. P., Siebenlist, K. R., Wall, J. S., Hainfeld, J. F. Evidence for a second type of fibril branch point in fibrin polymer networks, the trimolecular junction. *Blood,* 82:1517–1521, 1993.
7. Lorand, L., Conrad, S. M. Transglutaminases. *Molecular and Cellular Biochemistry,* 58:9–35, 1984.
8. Folk, J. E., Choong, I. S. Transglutaminases. *Methods Enzymol.*, 46:358–375, 1985.
9. Shainoff, J. R., Urbanic D. A., DiBello, P. M. Immunoelectrophoretic characterization of the cross-linking of fibrinogen and fibrin by factor XIIIa and tissue transglutaminase. *J. Biol. Chem.*, 266:6429–6437, 1991.
10. Preissner, K. T., Rotker, J., Scimayr, E., Fasold, H., Muller-Berghaus, G. Reversible interactions of fibrin and fibrinogen: An ultracentrifugation study. In: *Fibrinogen-Structural Variants and Interactions.* A. Henschen, B. Hessel, J. McDonagh, T. Saldeen, eds. Walter de Gruyter and Co., Berlin, p. 130–139, 1985.
11. Rotker, J., Preissner, K. T., Muller-Berghaus, G. Soluble fibrin consists of fibrin oligomers of heterogeneous distribution. *Eur. J. Biochem.*, 155:583–588, 1986.
12. Wilf, J., Minton, A. P. Soluble fibrin-fibrinogen complexes as intermediates in fibrin gel formation. *Biochemistry,* 25:3124–3133, 1986.
13. Husain, S. S., Weisel, J. W., Budzynski, A. Z. Interaction of fibrinogen and its derivative with fibrin. *J. Biol. Chem.*, 264:11414–11420, 1989.
14. Ferry, J. D. *Viscoelasticity of Polymers.* 3rd. ed. John Wiley and Sons, (NY), 1980.
15. Marx, G. Elasticity of fibrin and protofibrin gels is differentially modulated by calcium and zinc. *Thrombos Haemostas,* 59:500–503, 1988.
16. Marx, G., Blankenfeld, A. Kinetic and mechanical parameters of pure cryoprecipitate fibrin. *Blood Coag. and Fibrinolys.*, 4:73–78, 1992.

# *Chapter 7: Surgical Tissue Adhesives: Host Tissue Response, Adhesive Strength and Clinical Performance*

D. TORIUMI

## INTRODUCTION

The efficacy of surgical tissue adhesives can be evaluated in terms of host tissue response, adhesive strength, and clinical performance. This presentation will review several different methods for testing response and adhesive strength. The primary parameters for clinical performance include ease of use, clinical applications, and clinical need.

The type of testing method used to evaluate a particular adhesive is dependent on the properties of the adhesive. The cyanoacrylate derivatives demonstrate excellent binding strength, however, host tissue response is a major concern. Therefore, the cyanoacrylate derivatives are usually tested for tissue toxicity and not for binding strength. The fibrin tissue adhesives elicit minimal host tissue response but tend to have suboptimal adhesive strength. The fibrin tissue adhesives are usually tested for adhesive strength and effect on wound healing.

## HOST TISSUE RESPONSE TO ADHESIVES

Host tissue response to tissue adhesives can be tested using many different methods. It was preferable to use one of several animal models that quantitate the degree of host tissue response elicited by a surgical tissue adhesive. The rabbit ear model is one of the most sensitive animal models for testing host tissue toxicity [1–3]. In this model, a bone graft is harvested from the anterior wall of the frontal sinus in the rabbit. Then an incision is made in the thin skin overlying the ventral surface of the rabbit ear cartilage. After creating a small pocket, a drop of the tissue adhesive is placed between the bone graft and rabbit ear cartilage (Figure 7.1). After the adhesive polymerizes, the skin

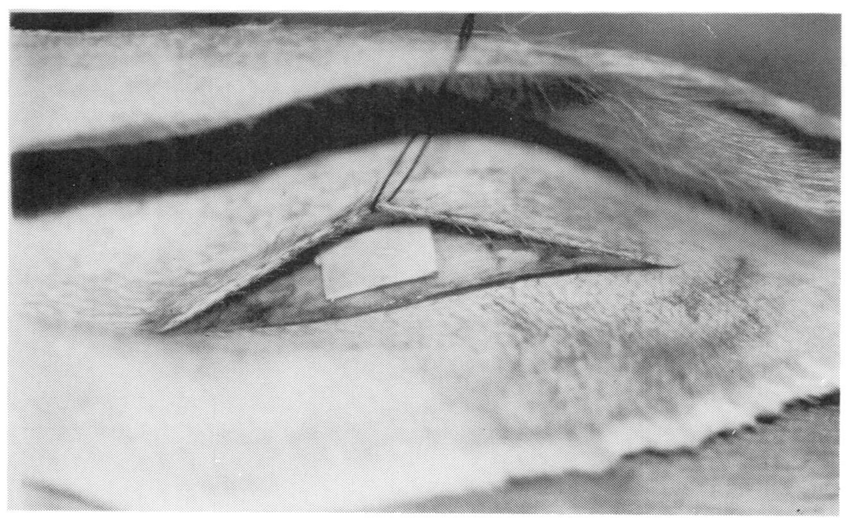

**FIGURE 7.1**
Bone graft glued to rabbit ear cartilage with a single drop of cyanoacrylate adhesive. After fixation of the graft, the thin skin of the rabbit ear was closed over the graft.

is closed over the bone graft. In another group of animals, a drop of tissue adhesive is placed on the ear cartilage with no bone graft. The thin skin of the rabbit ear is very sensitive to noxious materials and allows quantitation of the degree of inflammation exhibited by the adhesive.

After varying time periods ranging from three days to six months, the animals are sacrificed and the specimens harvested. The specimens are fixed in formalin, embedded, sectioned, and stained with hematoxylin and eosin. If a cyanoacrylate was used, oil red O stain is used to stain the polymer and to allow precise identification of the adhesive/host tissue interface [3]. Histomorphometric analysis is performed to quantitate the degree of acute and chronic inflammation by counting leukocytes and giant cells, respectively. The viability of the bone and cartilage are determined by examining the cellular morphology of the osteocytes and chondrocytes.

In a subsequent study using this model it was demonstrated that severe inflammation with ethyl cyanoacrylate resulted in necrosis of the bone graft and ear cartilage. There was minimal inflammation when butyl cyanoacrylate was implanted between the bone graft and ear cartilage [2]. In some cases the butyl cyanoacrylate polymer was extruded from between the graft and ear cartilage resulted in moderate inflammation. In a subsequent study, it was demonstrated that significant chronic inflammation occurred (foreign body giant cells) with butyl cyanoacrylate (Histoacryl®, Braun) when implanted on the rabbit ear cartilage without a bone graft [3].

Subcutaneous implantation of butyl cyanoacrylate polymer results in slow resorption releasing formaldehyde and cyanoacetate [4]. These toxic by-products result in acute inflammation and a chronic foreign body giant cell reaction. Many instances of prolonged inflammation, infection and extrusion of polymer occurred when butyl cyanoacrylate was implanted subcutaneously in the face (nose, ears, etc.). Both experimental and clinical findings suggest that presently available cyanoacrylate derivatives should not be used subcutaneously.

In another animal model, incisions of differing depths were made in pig skin followed by application of surgical tissue adhesives. In one study, incisions were made through epidermis, dermis, and muscle. The superficial incisions were covered with butyl cyanoacrylate. Butyl cyanoacrylate was implanted into the dermal and muscle incisions. After seven, fourteen, twenty-eight, and ninety days, the animals were sacrificed and the wounds harvested for analysis. After fixation, the specimens were embedded, sectioned, and stained. Histomorphometric analysis revealed no inflammation with the superficial incisions. Analysis of the dermal and muscle incisions revealed early acute inflammation followed by chronic foreign body giant cell reaction.

## BIOMECHANICAL TESTING OF ADHESIVES

Analysis of bonding strength can be performed using in vitro or in vivo testing. There is significant variability in tensile strength testing. To maximize validity of the testing, an Instron 4301 materials testing system was used. This type of testing system relies on precise instrumentation and complex electronics to provide reproducible testing. Stainless steel jigs were machined to precise specifications with a 2 cm by 2 cm adhesive surface [5,6]. Fresh, split-thickness pig skin was prepared with a Padgett dermatome and cut to fit the cyanoacrylate adhesive. With pig skin on both surfaces, different fibrin adhesive preparations were placed between the surfaces and allowed to polymerize. After a designated time, the jigs were placed into the testing system and pulled apart at a constant rate (Figure 7.2). The energy to failure was recorded for multiple samples to account for intersample variability.

Studies were performed on fibrin adhesive preparations of differing fibrinogen, thrombin, and Factor XIII concentrations. Many other variables, such as time of polymerization, temperature and relative concentrations of the different components were evaluated. Additionally, different

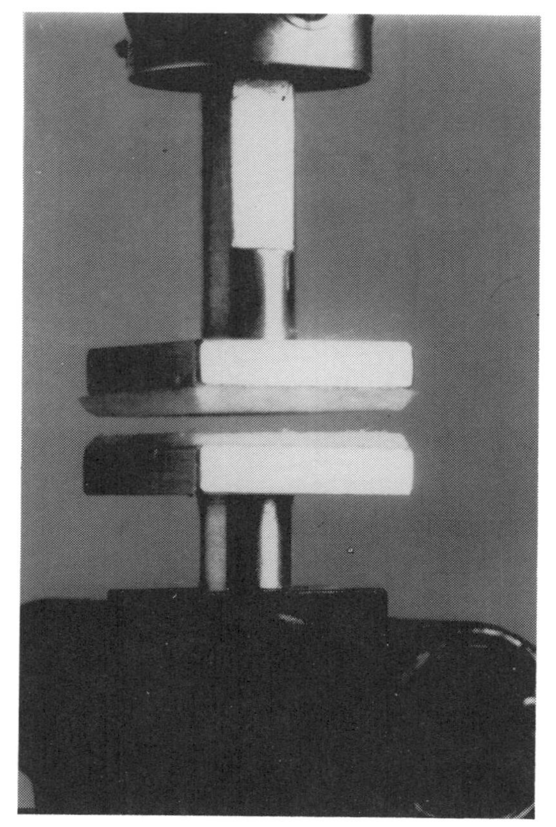

**FIGURE 7.2**
Stainless steel jigs with porcine skin grafts fixed to both testing surfaces. The fibrin adhesive was applied between these surfaces, allowed to polymerize, and pulled apart to failure using the Instron materials testing machine.

materials (fascia, etc.) were used on the surface of the jibs to change properties of the testing surface. Use of different testing surfaces allows evaluation of different adhesive/host tissue interfaces. The adhesive/host tissue interface is critical in the efficacy of the surgical adhesives. Adhesives tend not to bind to smooth, sebaceous surfaces, whereas adhesives tend to bind maximally to porous surfaces (fascia, periosteum, etc.).

Studies of fibrin tissue adhesives revealed that tensile strength was primarily dependent on fibrinogen concentration [6]. Maximal binding strengths were noted with fibrinogen concentrations between 40 mg/mL and 70 mg/mL. These high fibrinogen concentrations are difficult to attain using

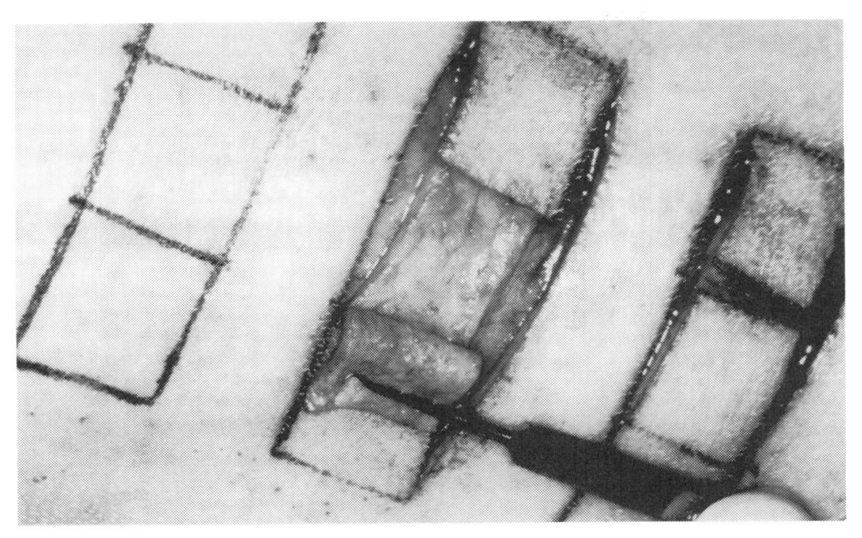

**FIGURE 7.3**
Elevation of 6 cm by 2 cm flaps in a pig model. The central 2 cm by 2 cm segment of the flap was split to create a bivalve overlapping segment.

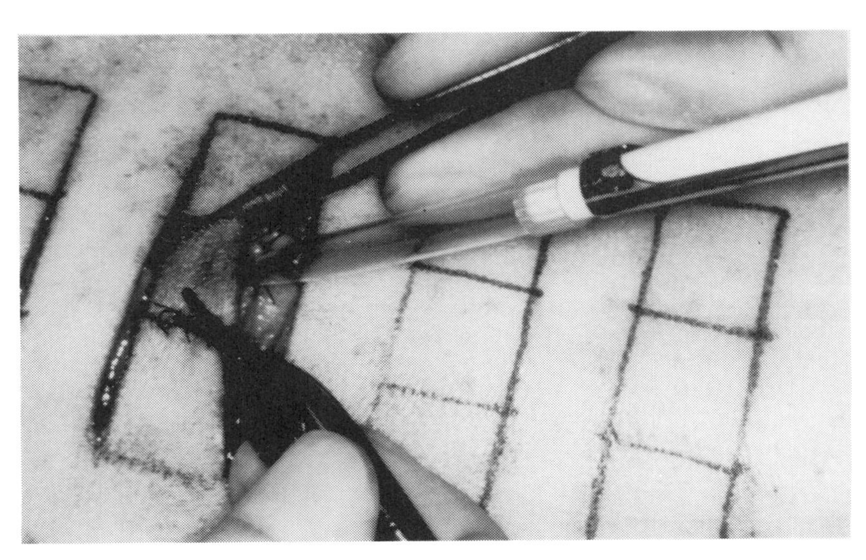

**FIGURE 7.4**
The adhesive to be tested was placed between the two central, overlapping segments and sutured to allow healing over a designated time.

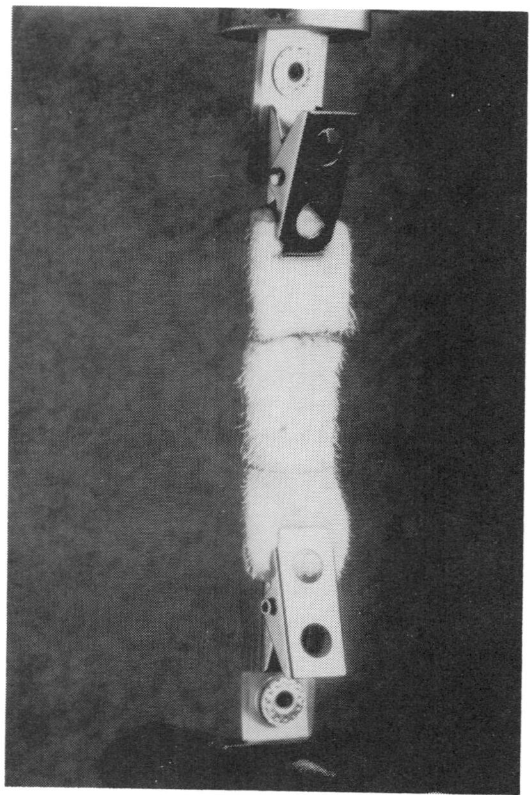

**FIGURE 7.5**
The flaps were harvested and fastened to jigs specially designed to fit the materials testing system. The flaps were pulled apart at a constant rate to assess the biomechanical strength of the overlapping segments.

standard methods of concentrating autologous fibrinogen (cryoprecipitation, alcohol, ammonium sulfate or ethylene glycol precipitation). Testing also demonstrated that thrombin concentrations are critical to the speed of polymerization. Concentrations of Factor XIII were found to be sufficient in the fibrinogen preparation and additional Factor XIII did not increase adhesive strength [7].

Adhesive strength can also be evaluated by using shear testing. In this animal model, 6 cm by 2 cm flaps were elevated in the subdermal plane along the flank of a pig. The flaps were divided into three 2 cm by 2 cm segments. The central 2 cm by 2 cm segment was split into a two-layer (bivalve) flap which overlaps (Figure 7.3). The adhesive to be tested was placed between the two overlapping flaps and sutured to prevent shear forces from acting on the adhesive bond (Figure 7.4). The flaps were allowed to heal for one, two, seven, fourteen, twenty-one, or twenty-eight days. After sacrificing the animals, the flaps were harvested and prepared for shear testing. After removing the sutures, the flaps were clamped into position and shear forces applied to failure (Figure 7.5).

This overlapping, pig-flap model tested the early shear strength of the adhesive as well as the effect of the adhesive on wound healing. During the first forty-eight hours, the adhesive provided increased strength to bond between the overlapping flaps. Shear forces between the flaps may result in disruption of the fibrin network that aids in wound healing (vascular ingrowth, collagen formation, etc.). Shear strength testing at seven and fourteen days tested the tensile strength of the wound and helped determine if the adhesive affects wound healing. Studies demonstrated improved wound strength within the first forty-eight hours. Wound strength between adhesive-treated wounds and untreated wounds were equivalent by twenty-one days.

Histologic analysis of cross sections taken through the overlapping pig flaps revealed rapid resorption of the fibrin adhesive within twenty-one days. If excessive adhesive was implanted between flaps, delayed healing with compromise in wound strength was demonstrated (Figure 7.6). Exces-

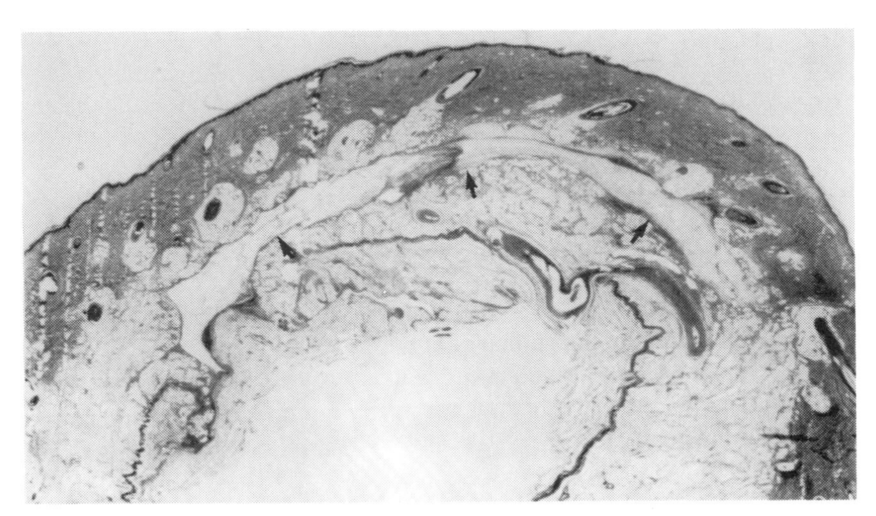

**FIGURE 7.6**
Microscopic exam of a cross section taken through the overlapping flap with fibrin adhesive at twenty-four hours. Note the excess adhesive that resulted in excess fibrin clot and compromised wound healing. Arrows point to fibrin clot between flaps (trichrome stain, lower power magnification).

sive fibrin adhesive can result in delayed vascularization, excessive fibrosis, or infection. When using fibrin adhesives, it is critical to use small quantities to avoid excessive clot formation between the flap surfaces. Application of a thin layer of adhesive at the adhesive/host tissue interface will maximize the effect of the adhesive and will not inhibit wound healing.

## CLINICAL EFFICACY

Surgical tissue adhesives are presently used for tissue bonding, tissue sealing, and hemostasis. In most cases of tissue bonding, adhesives are used in combination with sutures. This is due primarily to the lack of binding strength of adhesives presently used for tissue bonding. While cyanoacrylates possess excellent binding strength, tissue toxicity prohibits subcutaneous implantation. Cyanoacrylates can be used for epidermal skin closure if subcutaneous closure is secure and there is no tension on the epidermal closure. The edges of the epidermis should be opposed to prevent any leakage of cyanoacrylate adhesive into the wound. Cyanoacrylates can be used in combination with sutures to help seal the wound.

Fibrin tissue adhesives can be used for tissue sealing and hemostasis. Application of sutures to close a tear in the dura can create a larger defect. Fibrin adhesives can be used to bond fascia to a dural tear and help seal the cerebrospinal fluid leak. With this application, the strength of the adhesive is not as critical because the area of bonded surface is usually much greater than the size of the defect. Furthermore, the fibrin adhesive can act as a sealant to prevent leakage.

In some surgical procedures, bleeding from friable tissue (liver, lung, etc.) is difficult to manage. Cautery may result in increased tissue necrosis and suture ligation may result in further tissue damage. In these cases, fibrin based adhesives can be applied to the bleeding surface to slow or stop the bleeding by initiating the coagulation cascade.

Safety and ease of use are probably the most critical factors in the long-term success of surgical tissue adhesives. Safety issues will have to be determined by additional animal toxicity studies and clinical trials. Most surgeons will not use tissue adhesives if they are difficult to prepare and have suboptimal efficacy. In most cases, suture materials are effective in manipulation of tissues and wound closure. Surgeons will hesitate to alter conventional suture techniques for skin closure unless a surgical adhesive with properties superior to sutures is developed.

Surgical tissue adhesives may be useful in selected cases, such as in epidermal closure in children, by eliminating the need for suture removal. Application of skin grafts with fibrin tissue adhesive is popular because graft fixation is critical to survival. Graft survival can be increased by setting up a uniform fibrin network between the graft and host bed. This fibrin network acts as a scaffold for vascular ingrowth and collagen synthesis. The effect of shear forces acting on the graft can be minimized by the fibrin adhesive and help prevent disruption of the vascular supply to the graft.

## FINAL COMMENTS

In the future, a major use of tissue adhesives may be as a carrier vehicle for growth factors or other pharmaceutical agents. Fibrin adhesives resorb at a rapid rate and are already being used to deliver many types of growth factors. Fibrin adhesives composed of recombinant components will insure a safe, reproducible product that will surely have many clinical uses. New nontoxic forms of cyanoacrylate derivatives that resorb at a predictable rate may also prove to be an effective drug-delivery system. The future of surgical tissue adhesives will depend on the development of novel adhesive products with little host tissue response and improved performance.

## REFERENCES

1. Fung, R. O., Ronis, J. L., Mohr, R. M. Use of butyl-2-cyanoacrylate in rabbit auricular cartilage. *Arch. Otolaryngol.*, 111:459–464, 1985.
2. Toriumi, D. M., Raslan, W., Friedman, M., Tardy, M. E. Histotoxicity of cyanoacrylate tissue adhesives. *Arch. Otolaryngol. Head Neck Surg.*, 116:546–550, 1990.
3. Toriumi, D. M., Raslan, W., Friedman, M., Tardy, M. E. Variable histotoxicity of Histoacryl® when used in a subcutaneous site: An experimental study. *Laryngoscope,* 101:330–343, 1991.
4. Leonard, F., Kulkarni, R. K., Brandes, G., Nelson, J., Cameron, J. J. Synthesis and degradation of poly(alkyl-cyanoacrylates). *J. Appl. Polymer Sci.*, 10:259–272, 1966.
5. Sierra, D. H., Feldman, D., Saltz, R., Huang, S. A method to determine shear adhesive strength of fibrin sealants. *J. Appl. Biomat.*, 3:147–151, 1992.
6. Vogel, A., O'Grady, K., Toriumi, D. M. Surgical tissue adhesives in facial plastic and reconstructive surgery. *Fac. Plast. Surg. Monogr.*, 9:49–57, 1993.
7. Toriumi, D. M., Kotler, H., Walner, D., Geraghty, J. Investigation into increasing the binding strength of fibrin tissue adhesive. Presented at the Spring Meeting of the American Society of Head and Neck Surgery, Waikoloa, Hawaii, May 8, 1991.

# *Chapter 8: Biological and Rheological Properties of a Virally Inactivated Fibrin Glue (Biocol®): Comparison to an Autologous Fibrin Glue*

M. BURNOUF-RADOSEVICH, P. DUVAL, B. FLAN, P. APPOURCHAUX, C. MICHALSKI, T. BURNOUF and J. J. HUART

## INTRODUCTION

In the last two decades, several types of tissue adhesives have been developed to complement or substitute for sutures in surgical procedures. Some of them (e.g., cyanoacrylate derivatives) are of synthetic origin. They have high adhesive strength but poor biodegradable characteristics that often cause cytotoxicity and tissue necrosis. Other adhesives are of biological origin. Fibrin glues, for example, are products comprised of the purified plasma proteins that constitute the fibrin network. The latter structure, when formed with the right proportion of biologically active proteins, exhibits tissue compatibility, optimal hemostatic and healing properties as well as elasticity and relatively high adhesive strength.

However, early fibrin-glue preparations were made of crude fibrinogen concentrates not subjected to viral-inactivation treatments which avoid risks of viral transmission. These were not licensed in several countries, including the United States. This favored, particularly in the United States, the use of autologous fibrin glues that were prepared from the patient's own fibrinogen, but still depended on exogenous plasma proteins of animal origin (bovine thrombin) to induce clotting.

Fortunately, viral-inactivation/elimination techniques have evolved rapidly since it was learned that the AIDS virus could be transmitted by blood and plasma products. The solvent/detergent method first described by the New York Blood Center for a Factor VIII concentrate has been successfully applied to a fibrin glue manufactured in Europe since 1987 [1]. This method has proven its efficacy against lipid-enveloped viruses, a group that includes most of the life-threatening, plasma-borne viruses. Nonenveloped (N-E) viruses, such as hepatitis A and parvovirus B19, are of some concern, however, particularly in immunodeficient patients.

Additional techniques (e.g., dry-heat treatment, nanofiltration, etc.) are being evaluated in the production process of plasma-derived products to overcome the risks potentially associated with N-E viruses [2]. In addition to specific viral-inactivation treatments, purification procedures themselves may segregate viruses from therapeutic plasma proteins that improve the overall security against resistant viruses [3].

This is a description of the characteristics of virus-inactivated fibrin glue product (Biocol®) subjected to a solvent/detergent (SD) treatment. Data on virus reduction titers are presented. The biological and rheological properties of this concentrate are compared to those of an autologous fibrin glue preparation.

## FIBRIN GLUE PRODUCTION

Fibrin glue is produced from pooled human plasma subjected to a fractionation scheme facilitating the isolation of more than fifteen different therapeutic proteins. This product is made of two concentrates: one is a mixture of fibrinogen, Factor XIII (FXIII) and fibronectin; the other is a highly purified human thrombin. The first concentrate is recovered from 300 liters of plasma by a multistep ethanol fractionation procedure that includes an SD treatment using tri-*n*-butyl phosphate (TnBP) and Tween-80. Thrombin is purified by chromatography as a by-product of a Factor IX production scheme and is also subjected to an SD treatment. Both concentrates are poured into vials and freeze-dried.

Careful automatic monitoring of the production parameters ensures reproducibility in the properties of the products. In addition, a nanofiltration step on 35- and 15-nm filters is being evaluated as a specific viral elimination step. A similar nanofiltration procedure has been successfully applied to Factor IX and Factor XI concentrates with high protein recovery (>90%). Viral spiking experiments to validate the nanofiltration step have revealed complete removal of viral infectivity including for small viruses, e.g., bovine parvovirus [4].

The fibrinogen concentrate of Biocol® solubilizes in five to ten minutes at room temperature in an aprotinin solution while the calcium-containing thrombin preparation is reconstituted almost instantaneously in water. Each concentrate is presented in prefilled syringes of 0.5, 1, 2 and 5 mL. Mixing of these components with a double-syringe system reproduces the last step of the coagulation cascade leading to the formation of a fibrin network.

The autologous fibrin glue (AFG) was prepared from a single unit of blood donation, centrifuged to remove cellular components, and subjected to cryoprecipitation at $-20° \pm 1°C$. Plasma was then centrifuged to

***Table 8.1.*** *Biochemical and biological properties.*

| | **Biocol®** | **Autologous FG** |
|---|---|---|
| Total protein | 120 | 90 |
| Clottable fibrinogen (g/L) | 105 | 48 |
| Factor XIII activity (U/mL) | 10–30 | 7–12 |
| Human thrombin (NIH-U/mL) | 500 | 500[a] |
| Calcium chloride (mM) | 60 | 60[a] |
| Adhesive strength (g/cm²)[b] | 163 | 114 |

[a]Added to the AFG preparation.
[b]Determined in a mouse model using skin grafts.

separate cryosupernatant under controlled conditions of speed and temperature. The resulting cryoprecipitate paste, weighing 3.5 grams, was recovered from the plastic bag with a syringe under a sterile laminar flow hood. All experiments with the AFG were done using the human thrombin concentrate.

## BIOCHEMICAL AND BIOLOGICAL PROPERTIES

Table 8.1 summarizes the composition of this preparation as compared to AFG. The active principle in the fibrin glue is represented by clottable fibrinogen that in Biocol® is highly concentrated (105 g/l). Not surprisingly, AFG contained roughly half of this concentration (48 g/l) as a typical, well-controlled cryoprecipitate does. Purity, expressed as a percentage of total protein, was much higher for Biocol® (88%) than for AFG (53%). FXIII, a transglutaminase that catalyzes fibrin polymerization, is about twice as concentrated in Biocol® than for AFG, thus contributing to its elasticity and adhesive strength. The latter parameter, determined in a mouse model using skin grafts, was also significantly higher for Biocol® (163 g/cm$^2$) than for AFG (114 g/cm$^2$). This is a highly reproducible animal test with a standard deviation as low as 7%.

## RHEOLOGICAL PROPERTIES

The rheological properties were also very different for these two types of fibrin glue (Table 8.2). Biocol® has a much higher viscosity at 20°C and a more convenient gelification time, (seven seconds), allowing easier handling (i.e., lower risk of clogging application devices), than AFG (0.21

*Table 8.2. Rheological properties.*

| | Biocol® | Autologous FG |
|---|---|---|
| Viscosity at 20°C (mPa.s) | 107 | 27 |
| Gelification time (sec) | 7 | 0.21 |
| Breaking point (N/m²) | >6300 | 4000 |
| Elasticity vs time | elastic (+)[a] | elastic (−)[a] |
| Elasticity vs shear frequency | stable (+) | stable (−) |

[a]Determined after one minute.

second). The breaking strength of Biocol® was >6300 N/m² while AFG broke at 4000 N/m², suggesting a higher resistance by the former to the pressure exerted by biological fluid in vivo. Higher elasticity over time and against shear forces was also observed for the former fibrin glue (Figure 8.1).

The optimal rheological characteristics of Biocol® may be explained by

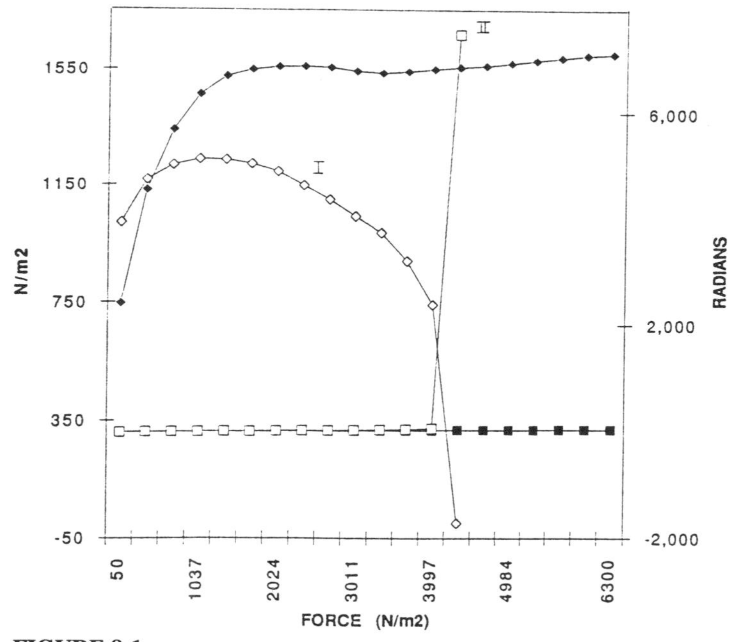


**FIGURE 8.1**
Rheological comparison of Biocol® and AFG. Breaking strength (squares): AFG (□) broke at point II. Biocol® (■) did not break at >6000 N/m². Elastic behavior (rhombi): AFT (◇) started losing elasticity at point I. Biocol® (◆) remained elastic.

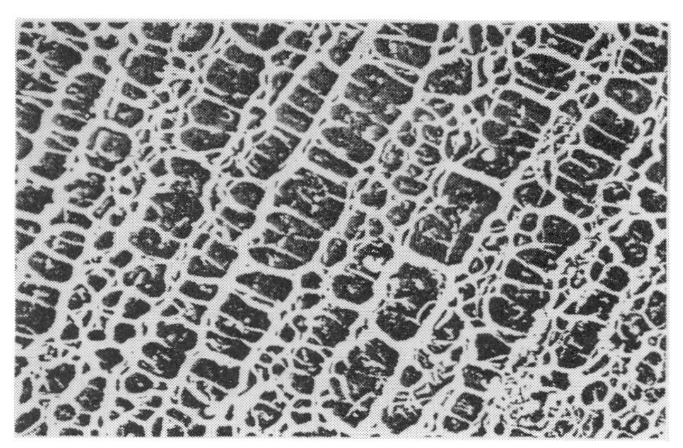

**FIGURE 8.2**
Fibrin clot ultrastructure of Biocol® showing a highly organized pore structure by scanning electron microscopy.

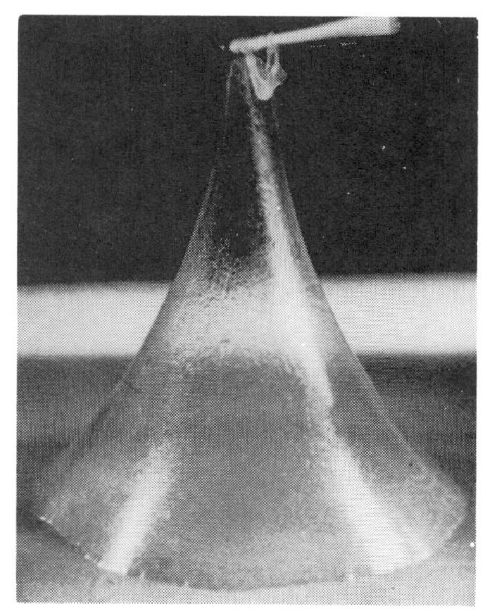

**FIGURE 8.3**
Fibrin clot elasticity observed ten seconds after spraying Biocol® components.

the highly organized structure of its fibrin network as revealed by scanning electron microscopy (Figure 8.2) resulting in a highly elastic and resistant fibrin clot (Figure 8.3) as opposed to the fibrin network obtained with an AFG (not shown) that was not well-structured, indicating a less elastic and resistant product.

## VIRAL SAFETY AND VALIDATION

Obviously, an essential point to consider when dealing with a product derived from pooled plasma is viral safety. Several procedures are applied to plasma products to control virus transmission (as performed by CRTS-Lille): (1) voluntary, unpaid plasma donations and donor selection to avoid high-risk populations; (2) viral screening of starting plasma for the absence of antibodies against anti-HIV-1 and -2, anti-HBc, and anti-HCV, anti-HTLV-2 and -2 as well as HBs antigen, and determination of the transaminase level; (4) viral inactivation treatments by solvent/detergent or pasteurization; (5) viral elimination procedures by nanofiltration.

The production process and the viral-inactivation method used for this fibrin glue were validated to demonstrate their respective efficacy in removing or inactivating viruses. Viral validation was done following the current European guidelines using host-relevant and model viruses: HIV-1, the AIDS virus; yellow fever virus (YFV), a model for hepatitis C virus; porcine pseudorabies virus (PRV), a model for herpes viruses; vesicular statitis virus (VSV) and sindbis virus, both good models for lipid-enveloped viruses showing medium-high resistance to virucidal treatments.

Viral-validation results (Table 8.3), obtained by independent laboratories including the Institute Pasteur in Paris, showed very high reduction factors for these viruses, e.g., more than 14.9 for HIV-1, and more than 10.6 for

***Table 8.3.*** *Viral validation of Biocol®. Total viral reduction factors (log 10) during the purification process and solvent/detergent treatment.*

| | Fibrinogen Concentrate | Thrombin Concentrate |
|---|---|---|
| HIV-1 | >14.9 | >10.1 |
| YFV | >10.6 | ND |
| PRV | >6.7 | >7.3 |
| VSV | >5 | ¢8.3 |
| Sindbis virus | >5.2 | ND |

ND: Nondetermined.

YFV during the production of the fibrinogen concentrate. A very high degree of safety was also obtained for these viruses during the manufacturing process of thrombin. These reduction values largely exceed the potential viral contamination of a plasma pool. In all cases, no residual viral infectivity was observed.

## CLINICAL APPLICATIONS

This preparation has been successfully used in general and abdominal surgery: visceral tears, partial hepatectomy, digestive anastomoses, fistulae repair, hemostasis of operatory cavities; in cardiac surgery: vascular protheses, aortic dissections, aneurysms; in stomatology: dental extractions in hemophiliacs; in oto-rhino-laryngology: repair of tympanic injuries, tonsillectomy; in neurosurgery: hemostasis of tumor excisions; in plastic surgery and microsurgery: cutaneous burn grafts, lifting, and blepharoplasties.

Its clinical efficacy was evidenced by the high hemostatic capacity as well as the rapid and aesthetic healing in the absence of sutures (e.g., skin grafts). This product was also shown to be an excellent support for grafted cells [5] or biomaterials and a promoter of angiogenesis as observed in the treatment of varicose veins and deep burns. Its tolerance has been demonstrated by the absence of side effects indicating its high degree of biocompatibility.

## REGULATORY ASPECTS

Biocol® was registered in France in 1984 and is undergoing registration in other countries. More than 350 liters of this fibrin glue have already been used in clinics in France corresponding to more than 100,000 clinical applications. The manufacturing process has a European and a U.S. patent issued [6].

## CONCLUSIONS

This fibrin glue preparation, due to its unique composition, represents a convenient and reproducible means of achieving effective hemostasis and healing without side effects.

As a product subjected to ethanol fractionation (fibrinogen), to chromatography (thrombin), and to specific viral-inactivation treatments, it has a high margin of viral safety against the major plasma-borne viruses. No viral transmission was reported in more than six years of clinical application.

Its rheological properties facilitate handling and improve its efficacy, particularly in some indications with a high risk of fistulae formation.

Contrary to autologous fibrin glue, Biocol® ensures reproducible behavior during surgical procedures and can be easily used with special application devices such as endoscopes and sprayers.

## REFERENCES


1. Burnouf-Radosevich, M., Burnouf, T., Huart, J. J. Biochemical and physical properties of a solvent detergent treated fibrin glue. *Vox Sang* 58:77–84, 1990.
2. Manmucci, P.M. Modern treatment of hemophilia: From the shadows towards the light. *Thromb. Haemostas.*, 70:117–123, 1993.
3. Burnouf, T. Chromatographic removal of viruses from plasma derivative. In: *Virological Safety Aspects of Plasma Derivatives*, F. Brown, ed. Karger, Basel. *Dev. Biol. Stand.*, 81:199–209, 1993.
4. Burnouf-Radosevich, M., Appourchaux, P., Huart, J. J., Burnouf, T. Nanofiltration, a new specific virus elimination method applied to high purity factor IX and factor XI concentrates. *Vox Sang* (in press, 1995).
5. Ronfard, V., Broly, H., Mitchell, V., Galizia J. P., Hochard, D., Chambon, E., Pellerin, P., Huart, J. J. Use of human keratinocytes cultured on fibrin glue in the treatment of burn wounds. *Burns*, 17:181–184, 1991.
6. Burnouf-Radosevich, M., Burnouf, T. Concentrate of thrombin-coagulable proteins, the method of obtaining same and therapeutical use thereof. U.S. patent 5,260,420, 1993.

# *Chapter 9: Assessment of Restored Tissue Elasticity in Prolonged in vivo Animal Tissue Healing: Comparing Fibrin Sealant to Suturing*

J. F. LONTZ, J. M. VERDERAMO, J. CAMAC, I. ARIKAN, D. ARIKAN and G. M. LEMOLE

## INTRODUCTION

The long-maintained interest in the use of fibrinogen concentrates in diverse clinical applications has been based on two prominent and distinctly different methods of preparation from plasma, namely, by (a) native cryoprecipitation in clinical preparations without any chemical intervention; and (b) chemical precipitation using saturated inorganic salts, notably ammonium sulfate, and organic admixtures with alcohol, amino acids, such as glycine, and polyethylene glycol [1–6].

The fibrin sealant emanates from the unique complex structure of the native soluble plasma protein fibrinogen comprising an intricate arrangement, shown in Figure 9.1, of three pairs of polypeptide chains ($\alpha$, $\beta$, $\gamma$) with two connecting three regions of more compact, complicated trinodular configurations. The native soluble intact molecular configurations depend upon an extensive series of hydrogen bonding along with numerous interchain and intrachain di-sulfhydryl (–S–S–) linkages of innumerable transient shifts into different configurations. This transient nature of native soluble fibrinogen is sensitive to exogenous changes in pH, ionic strength, and various inorganic salts and organic compounds that are used for preparing the precipitates of fibrinogen to varying degrees of solubility to incipient clotting.

The autologous native cryoprecipitated fibrinogen concentrates, produced under blood-bank standards, have yet to be assessed for effectiveness during in vivo tissue healing in terms of tissue strength and elasticity in order to complete restoration of biomechanical integrity. In turn, the reference standard would serve as the arbiter of chemically precipitated fibrinogen further processed by the sequence of lyophilization, storage, and reconstitution into fluid form with respect to maintaining or duplicating the

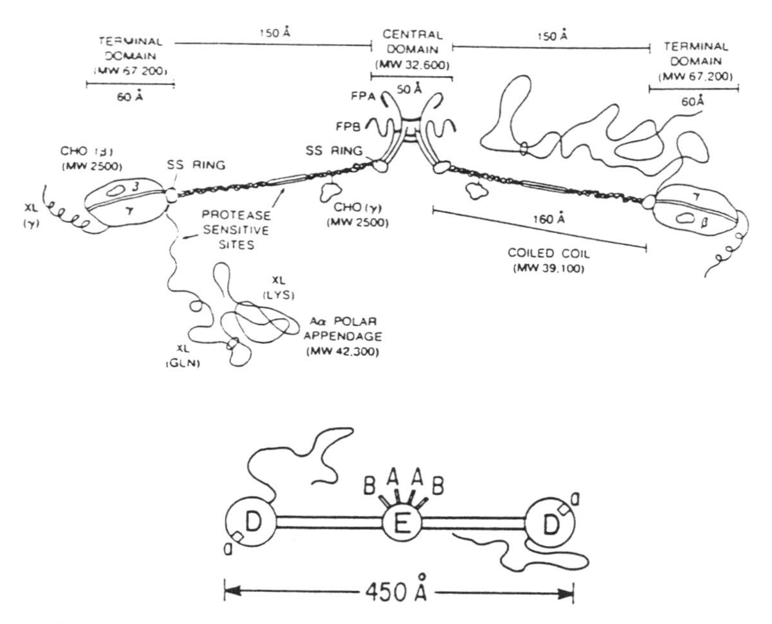


**FIGURE 9.1**
Schematic sketches of the fibrinogen molecule. Top: detailed structure showing the three pairs of polypeptide chains and the locations of binding sites, with two coil-coil, rodlike regions connecting three regions of more compact and complicated structure (reproduced with permission from Ref. [2] • 1984 by Annual Reviews Inc.). Bottom: abstraction of the above as two end nodules (D) and a central nodule (E) connected by rods. A, B (exact location not implied) denote fibrinopeptides split off by thrombin to uncover binding sites.

native intrinsic properties and extrinsic tissue bonding quality of the native cryoprecipitated form of fibrinogen [7].

The intrinsic properties relate to measurable constants of viscosity, adhesive tenacity, and the kinetic rates of the monomer formation, and polymerization with covalent cross-linking into fibril stranded configurations contribute to the ultimate in vivo biomechanical tissue structure [8]. The extent to which these native intrinsic properties and characteristics prevail in conversion to the lyophilized states and reconstituting of the extrinsic fibrin sealant quality has yet to be affirmed by in vivo mechanical evaluation. It is to this latter aspect of quality that the extended in vivo animal study of tissue restoration has been directed using cryoprecipitated fibrinogen concentrates to develop and provide a reference standard of selected measured tensile constants in the course of incision wound healing.

This reference standard, in turn, is compared to the measured tensile constants attained by conventional suturing.

This comparison is also believed compelling for the chemically precipitated, then lyophilized, and reconstituted aqueous fibrinogen products. There is the possibility that chemical incursion may deprive the fibrinogen and its associated protein of the unique native states and the proportionate components for cell growth and adhesive quality. This would be reflected in the course of the in vivo tissue healing from the applied tissue sealants. The associated plasma components comprise plasminogen, Factor XIII, fibronectin and immunoglobulins, which are cell growth factors essential to wound healing.

It is to this restoration of tissue healing, using cryoprecipitated native fibrinogen, that this presentation is directed. It illustrates a fibrin sealant reference standard compared to routine suture closure in an in vivo animal model. Tensile strength of the closure is measured over the course of wound healing.

The fibrin-sealant reference standard of this restricted presentation with specified test dimensions is intended to serve as a basis for the numerous other chemically variant precipitated fibrinogens, with further considerations of variables of adjustments in pH, ion concentrations, and imposed means of viral inactivation. The interaction of these variables can be expected to impose innumerable and unpredictable physical-chemical aberrations on the highly complex and labile configurations of native fibrinogen, which is readily prone to denaturation [9].

Although commercial lyophilized fibrin sealants from pooled plasma have attained widespread prominence, except in the United States, the need for monitoring safe and effective healing to restored biomechanical integrity by means of in vivo measured tensile strength and elasticity is still compelling for the assurance of safe and effective fibrin sealant quality.

## RESTORED BIOMECHANICAL TISSUE INTEGRITY

Physiological tissues are amenable to physical test measurements derivable from a typical stress-strain curve or profile such as depicted in Figure 9.2, also referred to as the load-extension curve.

The static stress-strain profile provides useful and meaningful connotations. Included are initial elasticity (a), often referred to as modulus, followed by the gradual increasing restraining slope (b), terminating as the ultimate tensile break force (c) at the corresponding ultimate elongation. These tensile characteristics with stated test dimensions provide measured constants for ascertaining the progress of the in vivo biomechanical wound

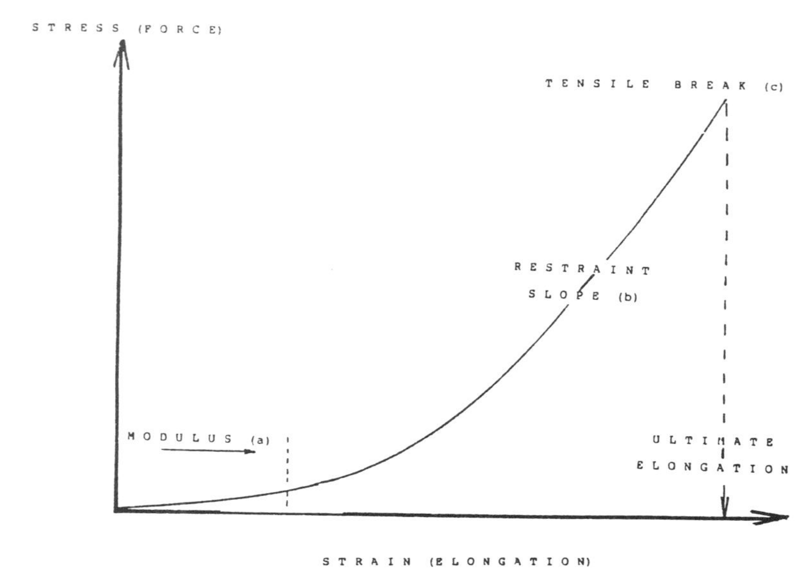


**FIGURE 9.2**

Stress-strain profile of rat dorsal skin retrieved from extended 90-day healing of incision closure with fibrin sealant starting from initial modulus (a) progressing through restraint (b) to tensile break (c) and ultimate elongation.

healing from initial fibrin bonding, through the ensuing critical healing to the ultimate restored tissue strength and elasticity.

This provides an important criteria for determining the in vivo effectiveness of the fibrinogen concentrate in wound healing of incised, repaired tissue, and this in turn can be expected to be dependent upon variables of preparation, whether by cryoprecipitation or by chemical precipitation, and the manner of activating the applied fibrin bonding mechanism. On this account, the tensile constants have been selected as an essential supplementary arbiter in comparing the progressive wound healing of native fibrinogen with sealants prepared either by cryoprecipitation or by chemical precipitation.

In support of the fibrin-sealant advances in structural tissue restoration, conventional histopathology provides an essential means for ascertaining healing during the course of cell growth and cell organization. It is, however, limited to subjective, qualitative, cellular observations. Qualitative assessment of cellular healing is valuable and provides during the in vivo animal tests additional affirmation of the restoration of normal static and dynamic stress and strain values [10]. In this study, the in vivo rat animal model is used for determining the tensile constants of healed fibrin sealant incisions compared to sutured incision closures on excised samples retrieved up to ninety days.

The data for study have been summarized in part previously and provide a rationale for the extended in vivo assessment for derived fibrin sealants by means of measured tensile strength and elasticity. This is to further enhance and exploit the surgical and hemostatic use of fibrin sealant in tissue reconstructions.

## MATERIALS AND METHODS

### Fibrin Sealant Preparations

Fibrinogen concentrates from fresh-frozen plasma stored at −20°C, or from cell-free, washed plasma separations, were prepared by a critically controlled thermal schedule from cryofreezing through thawing to centrifuging for maximum thermal diffusion. Proteins and factors associated with the precipitated fibrinogen include Factor XIII, fibronectin, transferrin, immunoglobulins, albumin, and prealbumins. These were substantially in proportion to that of corresponding initial plasma content as determined from polyacrylamide gel electrophoresis in both normal undissociated and dissociated sodium dodecylsulfate analyses.

The fibrinogen concentrates were produced from 38 mL lots of cryoprecipitated plasma in polypropylene centrifuge tubes, thawed, and centrifuged to produce from about 0.8 to 1.2 grams of a viscous fluid ranging up to 44% solids content. A nominal 24% (±2%) solids content was used in the present in vivo rat tensile retrieval series. The fibrinogen concentrates were generally used within eight hours of cryoprecipitation and could be stored at 0 to 4°C for at least several months without marked changes based on viscosity and surrogate ex vivo or ex anima tissue adhesion tests.

### Fibrin Sealant Application

For in vivo rat tissue sealing, 0.6 mL of the fibrinogen concentrate at the nominal 24% solids content was admixed in the polypropylene tube with 0.2 mL of freshly prepared solution of bovine thrombin (100 NIH units) in 1 mL of 40 mM calcium chloride by applying vibrational (Vortex Mixer) agitation for six to eight seconds. It was then applied immediately to the tissue sealant incision site. During the course of the in vivo rat fibrin sealant series, the 1.5/1 ratio of fibrinogen concentrate/thrombin solution (v/v) diluted the effective fibrinogen solids content by 40%.

## In vivo Animal Tissue Sealant Closures

Young Wistar rats, weighing initially 350 to 450 grams, were anesthetized with ketamine (35 mg/kg) and xylazine (5 mg/kg), shaved on the dorsal side bilaterally across the spine to a rectangular area 12 by 14 cm laterally across the spine, then scrubbed with povidone iodine solution. Two 6-cm, full-thickness incisions were made bilaterally 4 cm from the spine. One incision was sealed with fibrin glue midway (cm) with 7-0 proline. The other incision was closed using the 7-0 proline suture at approximately 2 mm intervals.

Both sutures were closed with an edged bandaged cover and the animal was belly banded for about a day. The animal was placed in a separate, isolated cage for the duration of the wound healing to avoid contact with other animals. The animals were sacrificed at six test periods of four, seven, fourteen, twenty-eight, sixty, and ninety days.

Retrieved rectangular sections of the healed wound closure areas of the test dorsal skin were retrieved, separated, and placed on a cutting board immersed in a mixture of serum and Ringer's solution. After preliminary comparisons of the tensile strength and elongation, replacement of the Ringer's serum mixture with plain sterile saline solution was found to provide substantially the same results in tensile strength and elasticity. The retrieved rectangular dorsal sections were cut in parallel lengths of approximately 12 mm widths across the fibrin sealant and suture closure line while still immersed in the solute or saline environment media. Thickness measurements made adjacent to, but not over to, the fibrin sealant or sutured line averaged 2.4 mm ± .001 mm in both directions. The cut tensile strips, still wet from immersion, were placed immediately between the tensile grips of the Instron Tensile Tester that was positioned in a clear plastic cup and immersed ($n = 4$) in the serum or saline (Figure 9.2).

## Tensile Constants—Measurements and Assessment

There is yet to be prescribed a standard procedure or protocol for measuring the tensile properties of living tissues, although tissue elasticity is an important distinguishing characteristic of various physiological tissues [11]. Since the structures of living tissue such as the muscle, skin, and hair skin are made up of polygeneric fiber-forming proteins, it is appropriate to borrow American Society of Testing and Materials (ASTM) test methods. The ASTM testing procedures include diverse polymeric materials such as plastic, rubber, and textile materials, as well as a special section on medical and surgical materials and devices [17].

Two methods were modified: test D412-83 for evaluating tensile rubber properties, and test D638-90 for tensile plastic properties. The dimensions of the skin specimens were within the test standard specifications. The test specimen dimensions averaged 2.4 mm in thickness, 1.27 cm width, and 2.54 cm initial extension length between grips. A strain rate of 5 cm per minute was used.

The tensile measurements were made on an Instron Tensile Tester (Model 1130), with the test specimens immersed in media in an open, clear plastic container, depicted in Figure 9.3a, where the bottom of the immersion container was fastened to the stationary base of the tensile tester. The test specimen was sandwiched between a pair of upper and lower acrylic grips, shown in Figure 9.3b, designed to prevent slippage of the test specimen during straining. The grit cloth was adhered by cyanoacrylate glue to 5 mm thick clear acrylic plate grips with four screw holes to secure the ends of the test specimens. The grips were provided with 3 mm insert holes through

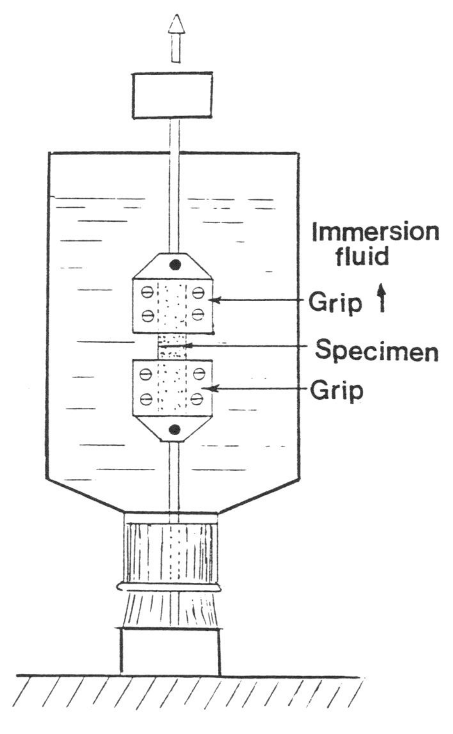


**FIGURE 9.3a**
Tensile testing total immersion system in a transparent bottle type container depicting emplacement of the retrieved healed rat skin specimen sandwiched between paired transparent acrylic upper and lower grips.

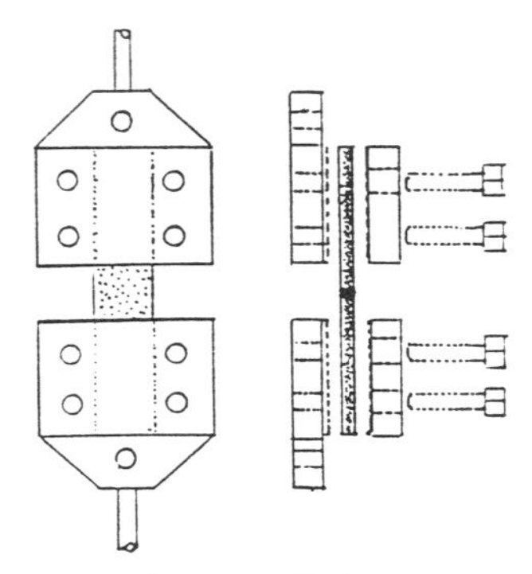


**FIGURE 9.3b**
Schematic front and side design views of tensile testing grips made of clear acrylic transparent plate surfaced with glued grit cloth to prevent slippage.

which 90° bent ends of 8 mm diameter rods were inserted for 5 to 10 mm length attachments to the lower stationary base and to the moving strain cell of the tensile tester.

The data were recorded as tensile force as a function of strain length. Figure 9.4 depicts stress-strain profiles of an early, critical, seven day

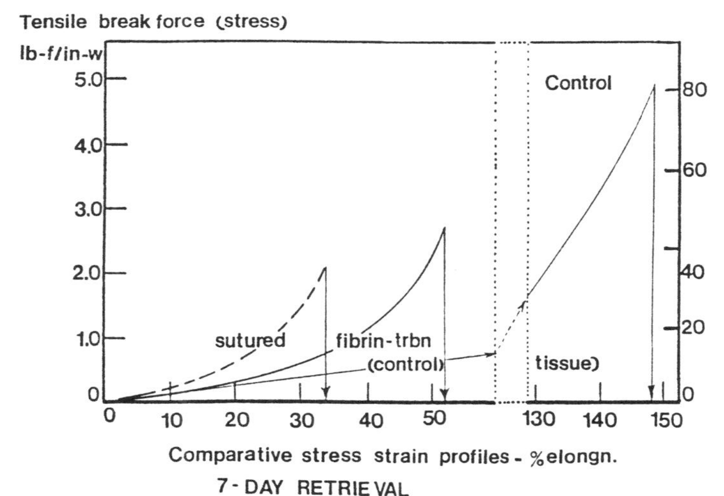


**FIGURE 9.4**
Comparing the early critical period of wound closure healing by means of stress-strain chart profile from which to measure the strength and elasticity of incision closure.

healing interval by comparing the tensile profile and fibrin and sutured closure to that of a nonincised control.

Each healed incision was tested with a minimum of quadruplicate test specimens (four to six) for each of the four, seven, fourteen, twenty-eight, sixty, and ninety-day healing intervals for both the fibrin sealant and the sutured wound closures. Nonincised test specimens cut adjacent to each end of the retrieved healed incisions were tested to provide measurement of intact tissue.

## RESULTS AND DISCUSSION

### Tensile Testing Results

The tensile data of the cryoprecipitated fibrin sealant are summarized in Table 9.1. These include static tensile break force, tensile strength, and percent of elongation when comparing fibrin-sealant bonding and conventional suturing. The static tensile modulus at the initial low elongations (10% to 20%) was 0.18 to 0.21 kg/cm²; the differences in all comparisons were unaffected by the rejoined incision to the bulk of the tissue. However, dynamic moduli measured by repetitive cyclic straining can be expected to reflect discernible differences among the three parameters.

### Tensile Break Strength

The control, nonincised specimens were from ninety-six rats with an average tensile break force of 2.24 kg/cm width, and with a standard deviation of ±5.19 (see Table 9.1). The tensile breaking strength, compared up to seven days, was not statistically significant despite the (−16.0 and −19.4%) differences between the fibrin sealant and the sutured closures.

***Table 9.1.*** *Comparison of tensile break force to failure. Sutured vs. fibrin-thrombin-$Ca^{2+}$ sealing. Units: kg/cm² (n test specimens).*

| | Retrieval–Days | | | | | |
|---|---|---|---|---|---|---|
| **Test Items** | **4** | **7** | **14** | **28** | **60** | **90** |
| Control | 13.65(41) | 14.71(41) | 13.96(48) | 14.44(51) | 16.17(51) | 13.92(5) |
| (a) Sutured | 0.104(4) | 0.386(4) | 0.738(5) | 2.770(5) | 8.649(6) | 8.763(5) |
| (b) Fibrin sealed | 0.089(4) | 0.461(4) | 0.949(5) | 3.306(5) | 9.292(6) | 14.56(5) |
| (c) Diff. ((b) − (a)) | −0.015 | 0.075 | 0.211 | 0.536 | 0.643 | 5.857 |
| (d) %((b) − (a)) | −14.0 | 16.3 | 22.1 | 16.2 | 6.92 | 40.2 |
| (e) Significance (*P*) | <0.05 | <0.01 | <0.001 | <0.01 | n/s | 0.001 |

The features of stress-strain characteristics serve to model the physiological dynamic straining [10]. This is particularly important in that only a fraction of elongation can be initially expended beyond which premature rupture or failure ensues. In this regard, the limits of elongation at each healing period can be useful in further assessing the basic matrix differences between the fibrin sealant and the sutured wound healing closures.

The fibrin sealant closures at fourteen days demonstrated substantially higher tensile break force, except at sixty days, attaining as much as 63.6% higher force than that of the sutured closure, which was approximately equivalent to that of the control. This illustrated a substantially complete restoration of biomechanical tissue integrity. Extrapolation of the extended sutured healing suggests complete healing would require an additional fifteen to thirty days.

## Tensile Strength

The break force is based on the width of the incision to which the fibrin sealant is applied or is sutured across which the strain or elongation is applied. Not taken into account is the equally important thickness dimension that provides the cross-sectional area. Accordingly, tensile strength measurement in terms of break force per unit area provides a definitive, common means for evaluating in vivo tissue healing.

As indicated in Table 9.2, the fibrin sealant provided higher tensile strength than that of healed sutured closures when compared for up to sixty days and followed by a significant increase (73.8%) over the sutured healing at the ninety-day retrieval. This represents nearly complete (95%) restoration of fibrin-sealant healed incision to the biomechanical integrity of the nonincised control.

## Tensile Elongation

Synonymous with the terms "stress" and "strain" is the implied measure of force resulting from the applied elongation. This is an indispensable criterion of failure often neglected in numerous published sources reporting on tensile strengths of tissue sealants. The evaluation of the extent of healed tissue elongations is important in static or dynamic testing.

As indicated in Table 9.3, the fibrin sealant at the seven-day period provided a significant increase in elongation over that of suturing. Finally, at ninety days, the fibrin sealant demonstrated a significant increase in elongation over the sutured closure. This was not the case, however, at the intermediate timepoints where sutured closures demonstrated higher elongation.

***Table 9.2.*** *Comparison of tensile modulus to failure. Sutured vs. fibrin-thrombin-$Ca^{2+}$ sealing. Units: $kg/cm^2$* (n *test specimens).*

| | Retrieval–Days | | | | | |
|---|---|---|---|---|---|---|
| **Test Items** | **4** | **7** | **14** | **28** | **60** | **90** |
| Control | – | 73.40(41) | 65.12(48) | 68.01(51) | 80.89(51) | 81.73(51) |
| (a) Sutured | 1.267(4) | 1.471(4) | 3.759(5) | 12.46(5) | 39.49(6) | 44.49(5) |
| (b) Fibrin sealed | 1.422(4) | 1.760(4) | 4.421(5) | 15.07(5) | 45.76(6) | 77.44(5) |
| (c) Diff. ((b)–(a)) | 0.155 | 0.289 | 0.662 | 2.61 | 6.27 | 32.95 |
| (d) % ((b)–(a)) | 10.8 | 16.4 | 15.0 | 17.3 | 13.7 | 42.6 |
| (e) Significance (*P*) | $<0.01$ | $<0.01$ | $<0.01$ | $<0.01$ | $<0.01$ | $<0.001$ |

The comparative merits of fibrin sealant over conventional suturing (e.g., higher tensile strength) constitute only a small portion of the numerous variables that could optimize the restored biomechanical integrity with either method of wound closure. For instance, in the case of suturing, the variable of materials, stitch intervals, lay of stitching, and other factors reasonably can be expected to moderate the comparison of the healing qualities.

The same can be said in the comparison of the tensile strength even though the fibrin-sealant closure was considerably higher than that of the sutured wound closure. But despite the significantly higher initial four-day elongation the two closures were comparable in the ensuing periods.

In conclusion, enhanced native fibrinogen concentrates prepared by cryoprecipitation were shown to be at least equivalent to conventional suturing in extended in vivo rat wound healing tests for tensile break strength and elasticity for restored biomechanical integrity. The measured tensile constants extending fully from the initial critical period provide a

***Table 9.3.*** *Comparison of tensile elongation to failure. Sutured vs. fibrin-thrombin-$Ca^{2+}$ sealing. Units: Percent (cm/cm × 100)* (n *test specimens).*

| | Retrieval–Days | | | | | |
|---|---|---|---|---|---|---|
| **Test Items** | **4** | **7** | **14** | **28** | **60** | **90** |
| Control | – | 149.3(41) | 177.1(48) | 149.2(51) | 136.1(51) | 124.5(51) |
| (a) Sutured | – | 33.2(4) | 50.6(5) | 72.5(5) | 98.5(6) | 94.0(5) |
| (b) Fibrin sealed | – | 52.3(4) | 42.4(5) | 68.7(5) | 86.8(6) | 113.0(5) |
| (c) Diff. ((b)–(a)) | – | +19.1 | –8.2 | –3.8 | –11.7 | +19.0 |
| (d) % ((b)–(a)) | – | +57.5 | –16.2 | –5.2 | –11.9 | +20.2 |
| (e) Significance (*P*) | – | $<0.001$ | n/s | n/s | n/s | $<0.01$ |

means for assessing comparable merits of process improvements not only with cryoprecipitation but also with other precipitating methods that may have cogent merits for clinical usage. The lyophilized, reconstituted fibrin sealants attest well as effective and successful replication of cryoprecipitated fibrin sealants but have problems of reconstitution time, delaying their ready use during surgery.

## REFERENCES


1. Schlag, O., Redl, H. *Fibrin Sealant in Operative Medicine.* Vol. 7, Springer-Verlag, New York, 1986.
2. Harker, L. A., Slichter, S. J. Platelet and fibrinogen consumption in man. *N. Eng. J. Med.*, 287:999–1005, 1972.
3. Wolf, G. Der konzentierte autologe gewebkleber. Paper presented at the Australian National ENT Congress, Oct. 1982.
4. Cohn, E. J., Strong, L. E., Hughes, Jr., W. L., Mulford, D. J., Ashworth, J. N., Melin, M., Taylor H. L. J. *J. Amer. Chem. Soc.*, 68:459, 1946.
5. Kazal, L. A., Amsel, S., Miller, O. P., Tocans, R. The preparation and some properties of human fibrinogen concentrations in man. *Pro. Soc. Exp. Bio. Med.*, 113:989–994, 1963.
6. Epstein, G. H., Weisman, R. A., Zwillenberg, S., Schreiber, A. D. A new autologous fibrinogen-based adhesive for otologic surgery. *Ann. Otol. Rhinol. Laryngol.*, 95:40–45, 1986. Also: Polson, A., Potgieter, G. H., Lazgier, J. F., Mears, G. E., Jaubert, F. S. The fractionation of protein mixtures by linear polymers of high molecular weight. *Biochem. Biophys. Acta,* 82:463–475, 1964.
7. Ferry, J. D., Morrison, P. R. Preparation and properties of serum and plasma proteins. VIII. The conversion of human fibrinogen to fibrin under various conditions. *J. Amer. Chem. Soc.*, 69:388–400, 1947.
8. Mosesson, M., Seibenlist, K. R., Amrani, D. L., DiOrio, J. Identification of covalently linked trimeric and tetrameric D domains in cross-linked fibrin. *Proc. Natl. Acad. Sci. USA,* 86:1113–1117, 1989.
9. Doolittle, R. F. *Fibrinogen and Fibrin. The Plasma Proteins,* vol. 2, second edition. F. W. Putnam, ed., pp. 118 and 133, Academic Press, New York, 1975.
10. Annual Book of Standards, Vol. 13.01. Medical Devices. American Society for Testing and Materials, Philadelphia, PA.
11. Lontz, J. F., Verderamo, J. M., Camac, J., Arikan, I., Arikan, D. Lemole, G. M. *Symposium on surgical tissue adhesives.* Directors, Saltz, R., Sierra, D., Atlanta, GA, October 8–10, 1993.

# Chapter 10: *Veterinary Hemaseel®: Ex vivo and in vivo Studies on Bovine Fibrin Sealant*

T. BRODNIEWICZ, T. BUI-KHAC, P. EMIRE,
K. RUDNICKA and M. NOWOTARSKI

## INTRODUCTION

Veterinary Hemaseel® consists of two components: a coagulation protein component containing mostly fibrinogen and a thrombin component. The coagulation protein component is obtained from freshly collected bovine blood, which is separated in the laboratory into plasma and blood-cell fractions. Following this, plasma is frozen at a temperature below −30°C in transfer bags for a minimum of twenty-four hours.

The plasma is then processed as described in a separate communication from this laboratory in order to obtain solvent/detergent (S/D) virus-inactivated, coagulation protein component [1]. The thrombin component, being also subjected to S/D treatment, is obtained from a crude, commercial thrombin preparation.

According to current data, this is the first S/D-treated fibrin sealant derived from bovine plasma. The preparation procedure of this veterinary product and its final characteristic are very similar to that obtained from human plasma. Therefore, the experience and knowledge gained from the in vivo and ex vivo studies of this bovine product are of great value. Certain properties of this veterinary fibrin sealant will be discussed here.

## ANIMAL SAFETY STUDIES

A rabbit-dermal-irritation study and acute toxicity studies on mice and guinea pigs were performed. For the rabbit-dermal-irritation study, 0.25 mL of the coagulation protein solution, immediately followed by 0.25 mL of thrombin solution, were applied on a test site of a shaved rabbit. A separate site was abraded. The observations were made on control, nontreated and treated sites at one, twenty-four, forty-eight, seventy-two hours and then at twenty-four-hour intervals for a period of eight days. No irritation was observed at any test site, intact or abraded, during the eight-day observation period.

To perform the acute toxicity study, 0.5 mL of the coagulation component, followed by 0.5 mL of thrombin solution, were injected intraperitoneally into mice. The study was also done on guinea pigs. In this case, 2.5 mL of thrombin solution were injected intraperitoneally. All animals appeared normal through the study and had gained weight by the end of the seven-day observation period. No gross pathological lesions were observed from necropsy. It was concluded that the product was nontoxic.

## ACUTE TOPICAL HAEMOSTASIS STUDIES

Fibrin formation is responsible for the haemostatic properties of the coagulation protein component and is instrumental in the adherence to adjacent tissues. The influence of different fibrinogen and thrombin concentrations on the haemostatic properties of the product were investigated.

### Formulation

Nine formulations of fibrin sealant were tested: coagulation protein solution containing 40 mg of fibrinogen combined with 200, 500, and 1000 NIH-U of thrombin; 70 mg of fibrinogen solution combined with 200, 500, 1000 NIH-U of thrombin; and 90 mg of fibrinogen solution combined with 200, 500, 1000 NIH-U of thrombin.

### Animal Model

The rabbit's marginal ear vein was chosen. In a screening study, a single transverse incision 5 mm in width and 1.5–2 mm deep was performed on both marginal veins. On one ear the mixed product was applied, while another ear acted as an untreated control. Pressure was not applied. Two parameters were monitored: bleeding time and collected blood volume. The results obtained were statistically different for the treated and non-treated ears and the haemostatic properties of the product (one-way ANOVA, $p < 0.05$).

To demonstrate more effectively the haemostatic properties of the preparation, an animal model was designed based on the following preliminary studies. Heparinized rabbits with 400 U/kg heparin were used and three combinations of coagulation proteins were tested: 40, 70, and 90 mg of fibrinogen each combined with 200 NIH-U of thrombin. Each of these

***Table 10.1.*** *Influence of different preparations on blood volume and bleeding time. In vivo studies.*

| Product (Fbgn/Throm.) | Amount of Blood Test (mL) | Amount of Blood Control (mL) | Bleeding Time Test (sec.) | Bleeding Time Control (sec.) | Forceps Used |
|---|---|---|---|---|---|
| 40 mg/ | 0.0 | 6.6 ± 2.5 | 0.0 | 256.0 ± 38 | yes |
| 200 NIH-U | 1.1 ± 0.1 | 6.9 ± 2.0 | 83.6 ± 28.4 | 253.0 ± 44 | no |
| 70 mg/l | 1.2 ± 1.0 | >10.7 ± 1.7 | 76.2 ± 73.4 | >240.6 ± 67 | yes |
| 200 NIH-U | 2.1 ± 1.6 | >8.5 ± 2.7 | 101.2 ± 70 | >225 ± 65 | no |
| 90 mg/ | 0.6 ± 1.4 | >9.4 ± 2.5 | 25.6 ± 57.2 | >217 ± 2.5 | yes |
| 200 NIH-U | 0.4 ± 0.5 | 5.6 ± 1.4 | 20.6 ± 38.8 | 155 ± 38.6 | no |

The results are mean with ±S.D. Each result is obtained from five animals.

three combinations was tested on ten animals, however, on five of the ten animals, forceps were used to stop the bleeding for forty-five seconds, and on another five animals the product was applied directly on bleeding wounds. In each case, the second ear of the animals always served as a control.

Blood volume and bleeding time were monitored and compared with the control of the same rabbit. It was concluded that product was an efficient haemostatic product even when a high level of anticoagulant was used. The results are presented in Table 10.1. There was an observed, statistically significant difference (ANOVA, one-way analysis of variance) between the test and control sites (at $p \leq 0.05$) for both time and volume for each of the combinations.

## IN VIVO STUDIES OF WOUND SEALING AND HEALING

### Preparation

For short-term study 1 (Table 10.2), 70 and 40 mg of fibrinogen were combined with 200 NIH-U of thrombin. The combinations of 70 mg of fibrinogen with 200 NIH-U and 400 NIH-U of thrombin were selected for short-term study 2 (Table 10.3) described below. The long-term study (Table 10.4) was designed to evaluate the healing process.

### Animal Model

A well-established rat model was selected. One, full-thickness cutaneous incision (6 cm long), which included the *panniculus carnosus,* was made longitudinally on the dorsal skin of the animals. The incision was immedi-

*Table 10.2. Tensile strength in vivo. Short-term study 1.*

| | Tensile Strength (Newtons) | |
|---|---|---|
| **Product Fbgn/Throm.** | **2 hours**[a] | **4 hours**[a] |
| Controls | 0.15 ± 0.03<br>($n$ = 5) | 0.13 ± 0.01<br>($n$ = 5) |
| 40 mg/200 NIH-U[b] | 0.69 ± 1.10[c]<br>($n$ = 8) | 0.64 ± 0.07[c]<br>($n$ = 8) |
| 70 mg/200 NIH-U[b] | 0.78 ± 0.14[c]<br>($n$ = 7) | 0.93 ± 0.18[c]<br>($n$ = 7) |

[a]Effect of time: $p = 0.835$.
[b]Effect of treatment: $p < 0.0001$.
[c]$p < 0.05$ when compared to control rats.
Control < 40 mg = 70 mg.
Data are mean ± S.E.M.
$n$ = Number of animals with a minimum of three strips evaluated.

ately closed with sutures placed 1 cm apart. Following the required amount of time, the dorsal skin of each rat was excised after rat sacrifice, and cut into three strips, each 1 cm wide and 5 cm long. Strips were placed between the clamps of tensile test machine (Instron Model 1011, Canton, MA) and the amount of force required to break the strip was recorded.

The aim of studies 1 and 2 of wound sealing was to evaluate the influence of the final combination of fibrin sealant on the tensile strength of the wound two and four hours following application. Results are presented in Tables 10.2 and 10.3. The long-term healing study (Table 10.4) was to evaluate

*Table 10.3. Tensile strength in vivo. Short-term study 2.*

| | Tensile Strength (Newtons) | |
|---|---|---|
| **Product Fbgn/Throm.** | **2 hours**[a] | **4 hours**[a] |
| Controls | 0.15 ± 0.01<br>($n$ = 7) | 0.17 ± 0.02<br>($n$ = 5) |
| 70 mg/200 NIH-U[b] | 1.42 ± 0.10[c]<br>($n$ = 8) | 1.47 ± 0.18[c]<br>($n$ = 6) |
| 70 mg/200 NIH-U[b] | 1.30 ± 0.15[c]<br>($n$ = 5) | 1.29 ± 0.19[c]<br>($n$ = 8) |

[a]Effect of time: $p = 0.851$.
[b]Effect of treatment: $p < 0.0001$.
[c]$p < 0.05$ when compared to control rats.
Control < 500 NIH-U = 200 NIH-U thrombin.
Data are mean ± S.E.M.
$n$ = Number of animals with a minimum of three strips evaluated.

***Table 10.4.*** *Tensile strength in vivo. Long-term study.*

| | **Tensile Strength (Newtons)** | |
|---|---|---|
| **Product Fbgn/Throm.** | **7 days**[a] | **14 days**[a] |
| Controls | 2.76 ± 0.21 ($n$ = 7) | 6.70 ± 0.47 ($n$ = 8) |
| 70 mg/200 NIH-U[b] | 2.93 ± 0.18[c] ($n$ = 6 ) | 7.84 ± 0.27[a] ($n$ = 8) |

[a]Effect of time: $p = 0.001$.
[b]Effect of treatment: $p = 0.05$.
[c]$p < 0.05$ when compared to control rats.
Data are mean ± S.E.M.

the wound, seven and fourteen days following the application, by measuring the tensile strength and by histological examination.

The results of studies 1 and 2 indicated that there was no time effect, i.e., wound breaking strengths from controls and treated wounds were identical at two or four hours postwounding, and that all fibrin sealant treatments significantly increased wound healing strength through a sealing effect.

There was no difference short-term between 40 and 70 mg/mL fibrinogen, suggesting that in the presence of 200 NIH-U/mL thrombin maximal short-term effect was already achieved with 40 mg/mL fibrinogen. It could not be excluded that 70 mg/mL might have had greater mid-term or long-term effects. Both 200 NIH-U/mL and 500 NIH-U/mL thrombin gave similar results, suggesting that in the presence of 70 mg/mL fibrinogen, maximal short-term effect was achieved with 200 NIH-U/mL thrombin.

The results obtained from the long-term healing study are presented in Table 10.4.

Multiple comparison tests revealed that fibrin-treated wounds were significantly stronger on day 14 (+17%, $p < 0.05$) but not on day 7 (+6%, $p > 0.05$). Histological evaluation seven days after the application revealed that fibrin was surrounded by inflammatory cells whose role was likely to digest fibrin. The process of resorption was apparently almost completed on day fourteen, since no residual fibrin was macroscopically observed at that time.

## EX VIVO STUDIES

It was important to establish certain adhesive strength parameters of the product, differently combined, by ex vivo evaluation that could be per-

***Table 10.5.*** *Breaking strength ex vivo.*

| Product Fbgn/Throm. | Breaking Strength (Newtons) 10 min | 30 min | 60 min |
|---|---|---|---|
| 40 mg/200 NIH-U | 0.88 ± 0.02 | 2.33 ± 0.28 | 6.60 ± 0.80 |
| 40 mg/500 NIH-U | 0.88 ± 0.02 | 1.45 ± 0.53 | 3.30 ± 0.50 |
| 70 mg/200 NIH-U | 1.83 ± 0.46 | 7.33 ± 1.60 | 13.23 ± 1.30 |
| 70 mg/500 NIH-U | 1.86 ± 0.53 | 4.80 ± 1.20 | 5.20 ± 0.56 |

The results are mean ± S.E.M.

formed in the laboratory. Diagonally cut, juvenile, pig skin pieces 1 cm long and 3 mm thick were used. Fibrin sealant formulations were applied and the edges were approximated for a controlled amount of time. The required force to break the glued pieces of skin was monitored by a tensile test machine (Ametek, Mansfield Green Div., Largo, FL). The results are presented in Table 10.5.

The preliminary data revealed that the breaking strength did not necessarily increase proportionally with fibrinogen or thrombin concentration. This is probably due to rapid coagulation of the product before approaching the wound edges.

## CONCLUSION

Data presented here, concluded from animal studies, demonstrate that veterinary fibrin sealant is a nontoxic and nonirritating product. The applied solvent/detergent technique improves viral safety. In vivo studies showed the product efficiently improves haemostasis. It may be also used as a short-term wound sealant by enhancing the healing process. It is important to note that fibrin sealant is not designed as a product to replace sutures, but as a product supporting them in terms of haemostasis and inflammation reduction.

## REFERENCE

1. Horowitz, B., Wiebe, M. E., Lippin, A., Stryker, M. H. Inactivation of viruses in labile blood derivatives. *Transfusion,* 25:516–522, 1985.

# SECTION III

# LABORATORY APPLICATIONS

# *Chapter 11: Wound Healing Applications of Fibrin Sealants*

D. FELDMAN

## INTRODUCTION

To best determine the usage of tissue adhesives, such as fibrin sealants, it is important to examine the types of implants and the advantages of fibrin as a biomaterial. Further, in order to use fibrin to its fullest, it is critical to determine the optimal implant design for each application. One way of determining optimal implant design is by developing a biocompatibility hierarchy.

Biocompatibility is the study of how the host affects the implant (corrosion, degradation, etc.) and how the implant affects the host (inflammation, etc.). By developing a ranking system of host responses and implant responses, the most biocompatible implant system can be determined and then designed for each application.

To develop a biocompatibility hierarchy it is important to understand how biocompatibility is determined. When implants were first developed, biocompatibility was defined as "a general term meaning capable of being implanted; causing no systemic toxic reaction; having no carcinogenic qualities; and whose local tissue response neither compromises function nor causes pain, swelling, or neurosis." This is the definition of an inert biomaterial. However, it only tells what an implant cannot do, not what it can. Also, over the years, as biomaterials research has moved from designing inert implants to biointegrated implants to bioactive implants, this definition has become less useful.

There are other ways of looking at biocompatibility. In the 1970s biocompatibility was described as an interfacial problem. The body sees the surface of the biomaterial, which can differ from the bulk of the material. This helped lead to the attention to surface analysis and characterization that is still a large part of biomaterials research today.

Others have described biocompatibility as what one wants to occur in a particular situation. For example, dandelions may grow in a garden. However, if the dandelions grow in the middle of a lawn they are weeds and have to be removed. Therefore, biocompatibility is dependent on the application of the term.

It is also dependent on location. Different tissues in the body respond differently to the same implant. The eye of a rabbit, for example, is used for toxicity testing because of its sensitivity to any type of irritation.

Biocompatibility is also dependent on time. An implant can be biocompatible for short-term applications, but not long-term ones. Also, an implant may trigger a "bad" response in the short-term in order to elicit a "good" response in the long-term.

Biocompatibility is also dependent on the animal model used. The goal is use in humans, but no animal can perfectly duplicate the human clinical response. In addition, each animal model elicits different responses. The approach, however, has been to optimize implant design, using one or more animal models in order to be at least close to the optimal clinical design for humans.

## BIOCOMPATIBILITY HIERARCHY

In order to develop a biocompatibility hierarchy, it is necessary to look at the possible responses. For biocompatibility, both implant and host responses need to be examined (Table 11.1). Biocompatibility is both a study of these responses and an assessment of whether these responses are "good" (biocompatible) or "bad" (poor biocompatibility).

An implant can be inert or can be modified in the biological environment. In many cases these modifications can be detrimental and lead to poor biocompatibility. However, in other cases these are the types of responses wanted and are actually part of the implant design. They are, thus, biocompatible. Inert implants are the most common type of implants on the market. Most implants, like artificial joints, are designed to serve a function and not be altered in any way.

***Table 11.1.*** *Biocompatible responses.*

| Implant | Host |
|---|---|
| Inert | Inert |
| Surface Active | Biointegration |
| Drug Delivery | Severe |
| Degradable | Regeneration |

***Table 11.2.*** *Biocompatibility hierarchy.*

| Implant | Host |
|---|---|
| Regeneration | Degradable |
| Integration | Bioactive |
| Minimal Inflammation | Inert |
| Inert | |

The implant, however, can be designed to be modified in vivo. For example, it can be "surface active," i.e., having a bioglass, calcium phosphate, or biochemically active surface that can stimulate an in vivo response. An example of this is hydroxyapatite-coated dental implants. The implant can also serve as a drug-delivery system of biochemical agents—wound dressings, for example, that can release antibiotics. Or the implant can serve its function and dissolve away, like degradable sutures. Similarly the implant can stimulate an inert host response or an active response. Again many of these responses can be detrimental, but many times they can be beneficial.

Most implants presently on the market are inert, like artificial joints. They perform a function with as little modification of the host as possible. In some cases, however, it is beneficial to have the implant integrated with the host. A porous implant can be used to trigger tissue ingrowth. A bioactive calcium phosphate surface can be used to obtain direct bone attachment. Both can be used to achieve better long-term stability.

Sometimes, however, a severe initial response is needed or desired to get a good long-term response. For example, some implants are used to stimulate a fibrous capsule that can later be used as a blood vessel or tendon sheath.

Finally, some implants are designed to trigger a regenerative response. Since bone is regenerative, fracture fixation systems, such as bone plates, are designed to heal fractures by regeneration.

Although biomaterials have come a long way, and many responses can be stimulated, they still are not capable of completely duplicating the structure and function of the part replaced. In addition, man-made materials will lose part of their function and properties over time and cannot "heal" like biological tissue. Therefore, the ultimate biocompatible response is for the implant to stimulate tissue regeneration and then degrade completely. If a biocompatibility hierarchy were established (Table 11.2), this response would be at the top. Sometimes, however, with the current technology the tissue cannot regenerate adequately so different options lower in the hierarchy can be selected.

For example, artificial hips are used in cases of severe arthritis or avascular necrosis. Present capabilities for regeneration of bone and cartilage are not sufficient to have a degradable regenerative implant. Therefore, a prosthesis is used to replace the joint surface and part of the femur and the acetabulum. Work, however, continues toward moving up the hierarchy. Original implants were designed to be as inert as possible—just perform the function and lead to as few problems as possible. Techniques to reduce implant breakdown and reduce inflammatory response continue today.

More recently, however, porous and bioactive (calcium phosphate coated) implants have been used to increase stabilization and prevent long-term failures. Additionally, work is ongoing to regenerate cartilage and large sections of bone. Although progress has been made, many technical problems, such as regenerating the appropriate macrostructure and microstructure of the joint, as well as long-term function, still need to be solved.

Sometimes the device function is needed and the implant cannot be degraded away. For example, catheters need to provide access from outside the body to inside (a percutaneous device), and, therefore, are not designed to degrade. However, biomaterials research has not moved the design up the hierarchy. Original implants were designed to transport blood, fluids, or drugs across the skin causing as little inflammation as possible. In an effort to reduce the inflammation and long-term infection problems, porous catheter cuffs have been used to allow the implant to become more integrated with the surrounding tissue. This has increased the life of these devices. However, infection is still a problem with these devices partly because the tissue that grows into the cuffs is not similar enough to the healthy, noninflamed surrounding tissue. Therefore, research continues toward the design of better porous implants to help regenerate the normal tissue seal seen around natural percutaneous structures, such as teeth.

A hierarchy can be established to help in implant design. The degradable regenerative response should be the first choice to look at and the inert response should be the last.

An important question then becomes: how good are we at regeneration (Table 11.3)? Tissue can either regenerate, grow larger to fill the space (hypertrophy), or use scar tissue to fill the space. Of the four tissue types (epithelium, muscle, nerve, and connective tissue), only epithelium is totally regenerative. Its regenerative ability, however, is not unlimited and requires assistance in some cases. For example, skin grafting is required in burn patients to speed the healing process and reduce secondary complication.

For muscle, the tissue usually scars or hypertrophies. There is evidence of smooth muscle regeneration in artificial blood vessels and artificial

***Table 11.3*** *Tissue regeneration.*

| | **Epithelium** | **Smooth** | **Skeletal** | **Nerve** | **Bone** | **Dermis** |
|---|---|---|---|---|---|---|
| Regeneration | X | some | ? | some | X | some |
| Hypertrophy | | X | X | | | |
| Scar | | X | X | X | | X |

bladder as well as in cell culture. Although there is some evidence of skeletal muscle mitosis, this tissue heals mostly by scarring.

For nerves, healing occurs mostly by scarring. Recently, however, nerves have been regenerated over distances close to 1 cm as well as being sutured together to regain some function.

For connective tissue, two tissues of interest are bone and dense connective tissue like that found in the dermis of skin. Bone is regenerative, but only up to a certain size. Dermis usually scars, but work with artificial skin has succeeded in restoring much of the structure and function.

Therefore, research in many disciplines has been concentrating on a better understanding of how to make these types of tissue heal more by regeneration and less by scarring. In biomaterials this research has centered on how implants can be used to enhance the regeneration process.

## RAMIFICATIONS IN IMPLANT DESIGN: FIBRIN SEALANTS

Another question then becomes: how are degradable regenerative implants designed? Progress has been made to develop bioactive materials by having the optimal biomaterial merged with the optimal bioactivity. These systems are tested and optimized in vitro and in vivo prior to clinical testing. This process can be called "biomaterial-enhanced regeneration." Optimal bioactivity would be to enhance and optimize regenerative healing by controlling the speed and completeness of tissue repair by modifications in the implant bioactivity.

This optimal biochemical activity needs to be coupled with a biomaterial scaffold selected to achieve the quickest and most complete regenerative response. The best scaffolds are ones that allow regenerative tissue ingrowth as the scaffold degrades. Therefore, optimization requires the appropriate implant porosity as well as the implant degradation rate. Additionally, since the biochemical activity will likely be incorporated into the implant, optimization of drug delivery rate is also important.

One example of how the biocompatibility hierarchy can be applied to implant design is in the area of skin research. The two main problems are skin ulcers and burns. For skin ulcers, the two main types are pressure ulcers and diabetic ulcers. The problem is the additional cost to the patient (both medical and lost wages) due to the long period of time for these skin wounds to heal and bed rest that is usually required for healing. Even with surgery, bed rest can last up to six weeks.

For second-degree burns and donor sites, the problem is also the speed of healing. For third degree burns, which are usually grafted, the problem is graft-take and supply of grafts in patients with a high percentage of burned body surface. Therefore, systems are needed to more quickly stimulate regeneration in open skin wounds as well as help in skin graft-take.

Using the hierarchy, a degradable regenerative system was chosen. In vitro optimization was done to help determine the appropriate growth factors with optimized release kinetics [1]. Additionally, in vitro studies were done to optimize the environment (oxygen) and determine the adhesive strength of fibrin for skin grafts (Figure 11.1) [2,3].

Acidic fibroblast growth factor (a-FGF) was chosen for bioactivity because of its angiogenic effect and stimulation of the key wound healing cells. Fibrin was chosen as the scaffold system because it can polymerize in situ, conform to the wound shape, serve as a drug-delivery system, has bioactivity, and can be useful for skin-graft attachment. Since a-FGF can be incorporated into the fibrin as it is polymerized, the growth factor may be trapped intrafibrillary. The release has been shown to be mostly by fibrin degradation. Therefore, the growth factor is only released by cellular phagocytosis and tied to the healing process, thus creating a biofeedback loop.

In vivo studies are currently under way to test the fibrin system in a partial-thickness wound model. In this model four wounds were created on the back of a rabbit. Each wound was treated differently: fibrin alone, a-FGF alone, fibrin/a-FGF, and a control. Although results are promising so far (Figure 11.2) current efforts are aimed at making a better fibrin scaffold by making it porous and modifying the growth factor release kinetics. Initial studies with a 12% porous matrix have shown the benefit in stimulation of angiogenesis and tissue ingrowth (Table 11.4) [4].

At present two clinical trials are being established using the fibrin based systems: one with pressure-ulcer patients and one with burn patients. For pressure ulcers the goal is to test a degradable regenerative dressing that can reduce or eliminate the need for surgery and decrease time of bed rest. Two fibrin/a-FGF systems will be used (one porous and one not porous) and will be compared to topical a-FGF (as used in other clinical studies) as well as standard treatments.

For burn patients, the goal is to improve the graft-take by speeding angiogenesis and getting better skin graft/bed juxtaposition. The fibrin matrix, both with and without a-FGF, will be compared to the standard treatment (stapled) within each patient. In addition, systemic growth hor-

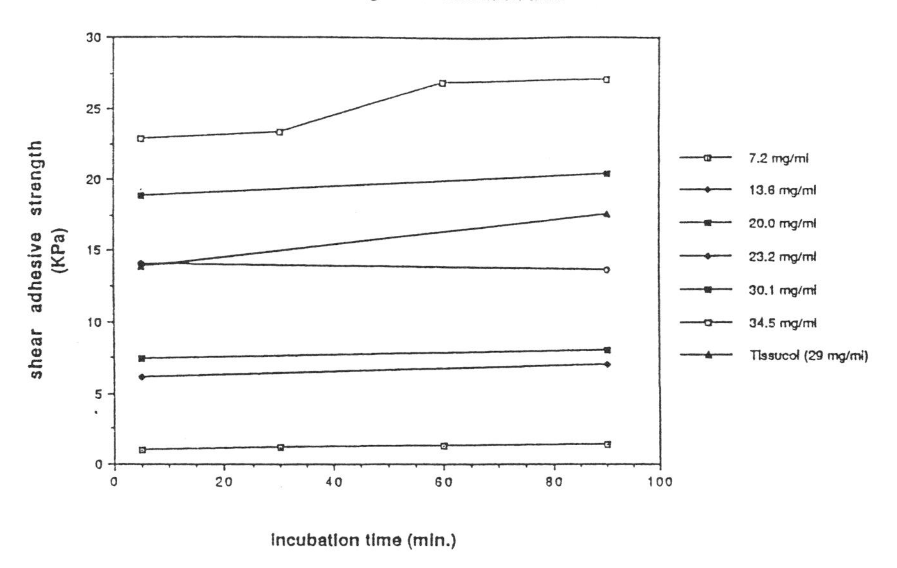


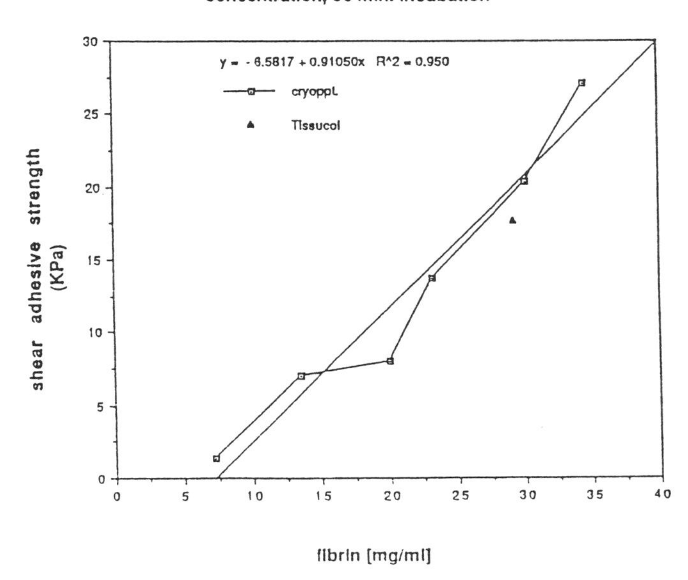


**FIGURE 11.1**
Ex vivo shear adhesive strength of FS as a function of fibrinogen concentration [2].

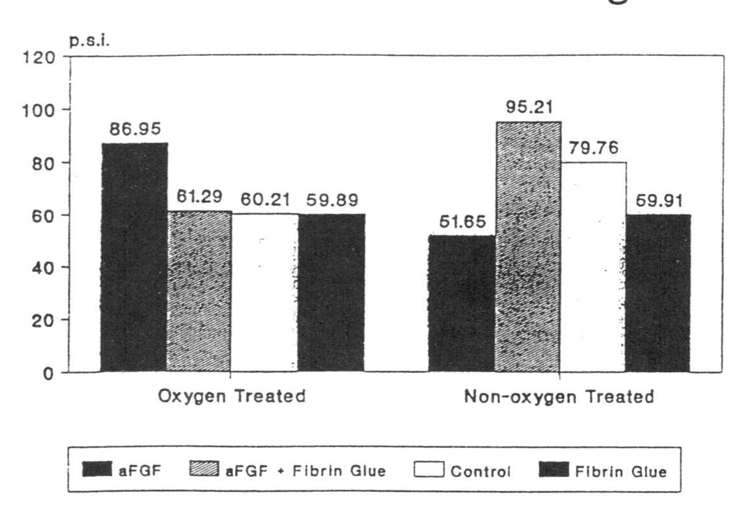


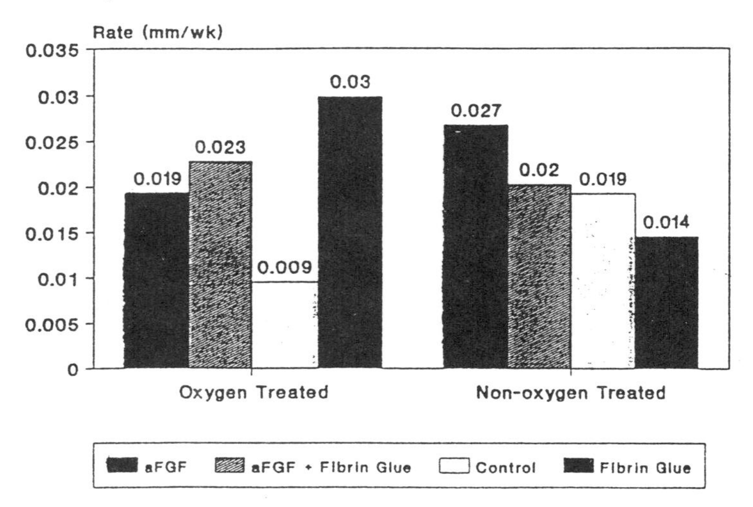


**FIGURE 11.2**
Fibrin/a-FGF tested in a rabbit model with and without 40% $O_2$ [5].

***Table 11.4.*** *Parameters of healing in a rabbit ear ulcer model after treatment with a porous and nonporous fibrin matrix [4].*

| Parameter | Location | Nonporous[a] | Porous[a] |
|---|---|---|---|
| Epithelialization rate mm/wk | | 1.73 ± 0.9 | 2.14 ± 0.7 |
| Contraction rate mm/wk | | 0.34 ± 0.46 | 0.62 ± 0.87 |
| Collagen (VF)% | center | 30.56 ± 4.3 | 30.33 ± 1.55 |
| | edge | 32.87 ± 5.92 | 38.06 ± 1.67[b] |
| Apparent blood vessel (VF)% | center | 1.57 ± 1.24 | 2.23 ± 1.67 |
| | edge | 1.57 ± 0.48 | 2.49 ± 1.58 |
| Number of blood vessel | center | 3.8 ± 1.53 | 8.65 ± 4.11 |
| | edge | 5.7 ± 0.95 | 11.31 ± 7.32 |

[a] $n = 5$.
[b] Indicates significant difference between the two treatment groups.
VF: Volume Fraction.

mone will be used on half the patients. This should help not only graft healing but also donor sites and second-degree burns.

Additional studies are currently under way using fibrin-based, drug-delivery systems for biomaterial enhanced regeneration of nerves, blood vessels, and bone [5,6]. Similar to the skin system of treatment, the fibrin serves not only as a biofeedback drug-delivery system for the growth factor, but also as a regenerative scaffold. Fibrin has many advantages that allow it to be used to help design biodegradable regenerative scaffolds for these as well as other applications.

## REFERENCES


1. Black, J. *Biological Performance of Materials: Fundamentals of Biocompatibility.* New York: Marcel Dekker, 1981.
2. Wilson, D., Feldman, D., Thompson, A. Fibrin glue as a matrix for a-FGF delivery in vivo. *Trans. Soc. Biomater.* 19:255, 1993.
3. Sierra, D., Feldman, D., Saltz, R., Huang, S. A method to determine the shear adhesive strength of fibrin sealants. *J. Appl. Biomater.*, 3:147–151, 1992.
4. Saltz, R., Sierra, D., Feldman, D., Saltz, M., Dimick, A., Vasconez, L. Experimental and clinical applications of fibrin glue. *Plast. Reconstr. Surg.*, 88:1005–1015, 1991.
5. Estridge, T., Feldman, D., Pandit, A., Andino, R. The effect of wound matrices on the healing of full-thickness defects in the rabbit model. *Trans. Soc. Biomater.*, 19:411, 1993.
6. Flahiff, C., Feldman, D., Saltz, R., Huang, S. Mechanical testing of fibrin adhesives for blood vessel anastomosis. *J. Biomat. Res.*, 26:481–491, 1992.
7. Flahiff, C., Blackwell, A., Feldman, D., Hollis, M. A degradable hierarchical composite for bone healing., *Trans. Soc. Biomater.*, 19:129, 1993.

# *Chapter 12: Fibrin Sealant: A Versatile Delivery Vehicle for Drugs and Biologics*

M. J. MacPHEE, M. P. SINGH, R. BRADY, JR., N. AKHYANI, G. LIAU, C. LASA, JR., C. HUE, A. BEST and W. DROHAN

## INTRODUCTION

The use of local delivery of drugs and biologics is expected to be beneficial in clinical situations in which there is ready access to the site to be treated, in which systemic therapy is either ineffective or produces burdensome side effects, or when systemic therapy is ineffective due to dose-limiting side effects. In these settings, local delivery formulations must have several characteristics. The formulation must be implantable in a manner that renders it immobile so that the matrix cannot "wander" or be dispersed to unintended locations.

If the material is to be implanted into tissue, as opposed to on the tissue, then the formulation should promote hemostasis in order to minimize undesirable sequelae arising from the implantation procedure. This will also minimize the possibility of the matrix being dispersed or of the medication being "flushed out" by local bleeding. The matrix must provide for appropriate delivery kinetics for the drug/biologic.

Finally, the matrix must be benign and not provoke an excessive or undesirable reaction from the body. Since few drugs or biologics have these inherent properties, most therapeutic compounds must be delivered in some form of carrier matrix.

The use of natural delivery matrices could be said to have its origins in Asia several thousand years ago when fibrin, in the form of powdered scabs, was used to deliver viruses for inoculation via the intranasal route. In modern times, three main groups of natural matrices have been the subject of research: collagen, chitin and its derivatives, and fibrin. Collagen has been used extensively in applications designed to heal damage to both soft [1] and hard [2] tissues, and chitin has been used to deliver antibiotics. Both collagen and chitin meet most of the previously mentioned criteria for delivery vehicles to some degree.

In contrast, fibrin excels in the first three areas of concern. Fibrin is recognized in most of the world as being one of the most effective hemostatic agents available [3]. It is used in Europe, Canada and Japan as a hemostatic agent and surgical adhesive [4]. Fibrin is found at the site of virtually all tissue injury and is broken down and replaced by healing tissue as part of the body's natural healing process. The ability to control bleeding, to remain firmly fixed in place, and to be naturally biodegradable has also made fibrin a good candidate for a delivery vehicle for the local administration of drugs. For these reasons, it would appear that fibrin is as desirable as a delivery vehicle as collagen and chitin and may have some superior characteristics.

It remains to be demonstrated that fibrin can act to deliver drugs and biologics with kinetics suitable for therapeutic applications. This chapter will summarize research experience using a commercial pooled fibrin sealant (FS) (American Red Cross, Rockville, MD) as the delivery vehicle, both in vitro and in vivo, for several drugs and biologics.

## ANTIBIOTIC DELIVERY FROM FIBRIN SEALANT

One of the first applications of fibrin as a matrix for drug delivery was its use in the delivery of antibiotics. European researchers, drawing upon their clinical experience with commercial pooled FS products, reasoned that there were many situations in which it would be desirable to also deliver antibiotics locally to prevent infection [5]. These researchers and others were unable to produce delivery kinetics of sufficient duration to be clinically useful [5–9], and this application was not pursued.

Using a novel approach to the formulation of the antibiotic, in vitro delivery times of over a month have been accomplished [10]. In the experiment shown in Figure 12.1, the antibiotics ciprofloxacine (CIP) and ampicillin (AMP) were incorporated in the anhydrous state into fibrin-sealant disks that were placed in 2 mL of PBS that was exchanged daily. The concentration of CIP in the eluates was measured using spectrophotometry at 340 nm. The quantitation of ampicillin in the eluted PBS was performed using bicinchonic acid (BCA) protein reagent and measured at 560 nm after complex formation.

For the case of ciprofloxacin, an initial burst of 8 mg (eluate concentration: 4 mg/mL) was found that declined exponentially with time. The release plateaued at 300 to 400 μg/mL after four days and remained in that range for at least fourteen days. For the case of ampicillin, the release had an initial burst of 18 mg (eluate concentration: 9 mg/mL) that declined dramatically

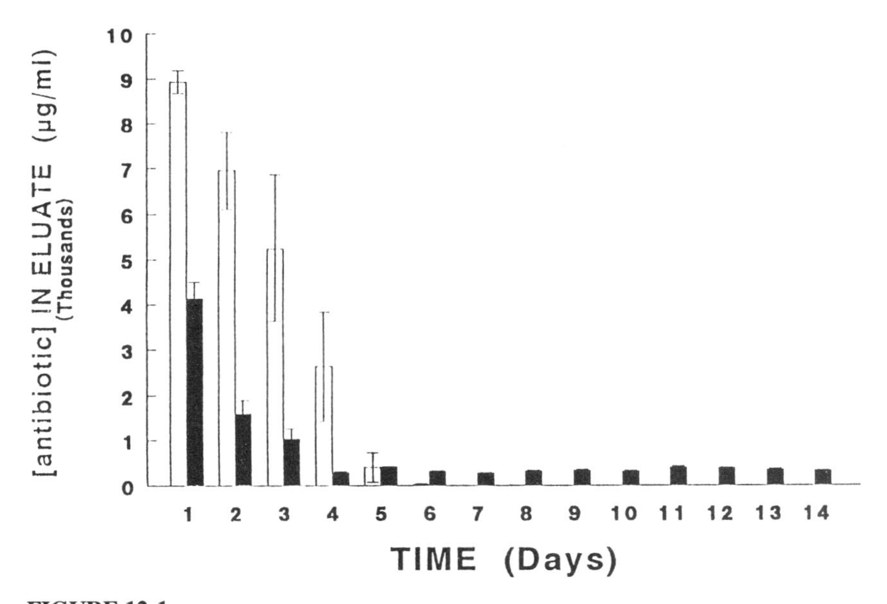


**FIGURE 12.1**
Delivery of ciprofloxacine and ampicillin from fibrin sealant. Anhydrous ciprofloxacine (CIP, open bars) or anhydrous ampicillin (AMP, solid bars) was incorporated into FS at a concentration of 345 mg/mL. The resulting mixtures were used to form discs 6 mm in diameter and approximately 2.3 mm thick. These discs were then placed in 2 mL of phosphate buffered saline (PBS) and incubated at 37°C. The PBS was exchanged daily and the concentration of CIP in the resulting eluates determined by spectrophotometry at 275 nm. The concentration of AMP in the eluates was determined using the BCA protein reagent and measured at 560 nm after complex formation.

with time. However, even after five days the eluate concentrations remained greater than 100 μg/mL. These results indicate that it is feasible to use antibiotic-supplemented fibrin sealants for the treatment of local or systemic infections.

In vitro experiments on the delivery of tetracycline from fibrin sealant resulted in delivery periods up to six weeks. Preliminary experiments suggest that these extended delivery periods, predicted by the in vitro modeling, also occur in vivo, and that similar antibiotic-FS formulations may be able to protect animals against lethal sepsis. The effect of other system parameters, such as fibrinogen concentration and antibiotic concentration, have also been studied. These experiments have indicated that the rate of release of tetracycline is independent on the fibrinogen concentration in the fibrin sealant and depends instead upon the amount of tetracycline loaded. A more complete description of this research is given elsewhere in this volume [10]. Antibiotic delivery from FS has been achieved for extended periods at concentrations that are considered clinically effective.

## DELIVERY OF CHEMOTHERAPEUTICS FROM FIBRIN SEALANT

Another area of interest is the local/regional delivery of chemotherapeutics to treat cancer. Researchers have shown significant preclinical [11] and clinical [12] efficacy in the treatment of cancerous lesions with 5-Fluorouracil (5-FU) delivered in a collagenous matrix. With the added benefits of its exceptional hemostatic and adhesive properties, it is believed that, in some situations, fibrin sealant may be a more desirable delivery vehicle for chemotherapeutics. Studies with 5-FU are described elsewhere in this book [13]. These results with 5-FU led to the consideration of other therapeutic compounds.

Recently, paclitaxel, or "Taxol," has been recognized as a very promising agent for the treatment of ovarian and breast cancers [14–16]. One problem with administering Taxol systemically is that it is highly insoluble in aqueous solutions. This has necessitated the use of a systemic delivery vehicle consisting of an oil and alcohol mixture [16]. This systemic delivery vehicle causes severe reactions in many patients, and current therapeutic applications call for premedication to minimize them [17,18]. The malignancies for which Taxol is currently used clinically are generally slow-growing, and it is thought that an extended exposure to Taxol would be desirable.

It has been demonstrated that the use of anhydrous [13] and, preferably, highly insoluble [14] forms of therapeutics result in prolonged delivery of the medication from FS. Additionally, the lesions produced by these diseases are often accessible clinically through percutaneous biopsy or laparoscopic procedures. Therefore, it was thought that the prolonged delivery of effective local concentrations of Taxol would be a desirable therapeutic goal and that FS would be an excellent delivery matrix for this drug.

The kinetics of Taxol delivery from FS were evaluated by first dissolving the compound using ethanol or the solid form, in order to incorporate it into a FS matrix that was subsequently placed into a histidine containing buffer. The buffer was incubated at 37°C and replaced every two days for a total of twelve days. The resulting eluates were then diluted and added at various concentrations to cultures of the human ovarian carcinoma cell line OVCAR, which were allowed to grow for five days. After the five-day period, the number of cells in each well was measured using the MTT assay (for further details see Chapter 15 in this volume [13]). In this assay, the

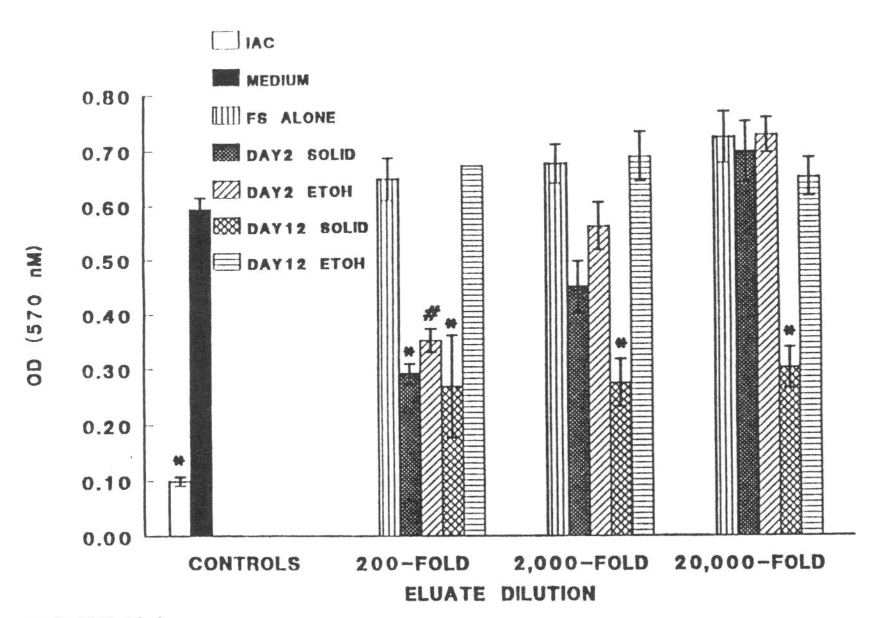


**FIGURE 12.2**
Delivery of taxol from fibrin sealant. An amount (0.26 mg) of Taxol, either in the anhydrous (SOLID) form or in solution in ethanol (ETOH), was incorporated into 400 μL of FS. The resulting clots were then placed in 2 mL of buffer and incubated at 37°C. The buffer was exchanged after two days and again ten days later. The relative concentration of Taxol in the resulting eluates was determined by measuring their ability to inhibit the growth of a human ovarian carcinoma cell line (OVCAR) in vitro. This assay was performed essentially as described elsewhere in this volume [13]. Briefly, 1000 OVCAR cells in 100 μL of growth medium were plated into each well of a ninety-six well culture plate and incubated for twenty-four hours. A 100 μL volume of various dilutions of the eluates was then placed into the wells (ten wells per dilution) and the plates incubated at 37°C. After five days the number of cells in each well was measured using the MTT assay as detailed elsewhere [13]. Controls included the addition of medium alone (MEDIUM) and medium that came from supernatants of wells containing only FS (FS ALONE). The assay was also performed on ten wells containing only OVCAR cells on the day that the supernatants were added in order to determine the initial MTT-reducing activity of the OVCAR cells at the beginning of the assay (IAC). The source of each eluate is given in the legend on the figure (*: $p < .001$ and #: $p < .05$ relative to the medium control (Dunn's test).

effect of an antiproliferative agent is to decrease the number of cells in the final cultures and, consequently, to decrease the amount of MTT that is converted into a chromophore detected by spectrophotometry at 570 nm.

The results of the experiment are shown in Figure 12.2. The controls included an initial (cellular) activity control (IAC), showing the amount of substrate produced by the OVCAR cells at the time of addition of the eluates, and the medium control, showing the maximum amount of substrate produced after five days in culture. The eluates from FS alone did not affect this growth. When Taxol was incorporated into the FS in the solid anhydrous form, the OVCAR cells were significantly inhibited by the two-day eluates at dilutions of 1:200 and 1:2000. Subsequent eluates recovered after an additional ten days in culture (day 12 eluates) also significantly inhibited the growth of OVCAR cells at dilutions from 1:200 to 1:20,000. This indicated that delivery continued beyond the initial two-day period and that the amount of Taxol delivered in the period from day 2 to day 12 exceeded the amount delivered in the first forty-eight hours.

The results obtained using Taxol in solution in ethanol showed that it was completely delivered within the first twelve days as these supernatants significantly inhibited the growth of OVCAR cells at low dilution. However, the subsequent supernatant collected after twelve days showed no growth inhibition. These results demonstrate that delivery of Taxol from FS for short or extended periods is feasible. More detailed experiments, both in vitro and in vivo, are under way to continue the development of this therapeutic application.

## FIBRIN SEALANT AS A DELIVERY VEHICLE FOR OSTEOINDUCERS

Another area of research has been the use of FS as a delivery vehicle for osteoinductive substances. These have included demineralized bone powder and bone morphogenetic proteins (BMPs). The results obtained from the delivery of purified bovine BMP-3 from FS are shown in Figure 12.3. The use of FS as the delivery vehicle resulted in the generation of osteoid matrix and was compatible with bone formation. In other experiments it was demonstrated that FS can be used to deliver bone-inducing, demineralized bone powder to both bony and nonbony sites. The result was trabecular bone formation in the desired location and shape of the implant. A more detailed description of work involving the use of FS as a delivery vehicle for bone inducing substances can be found in this volume [4].

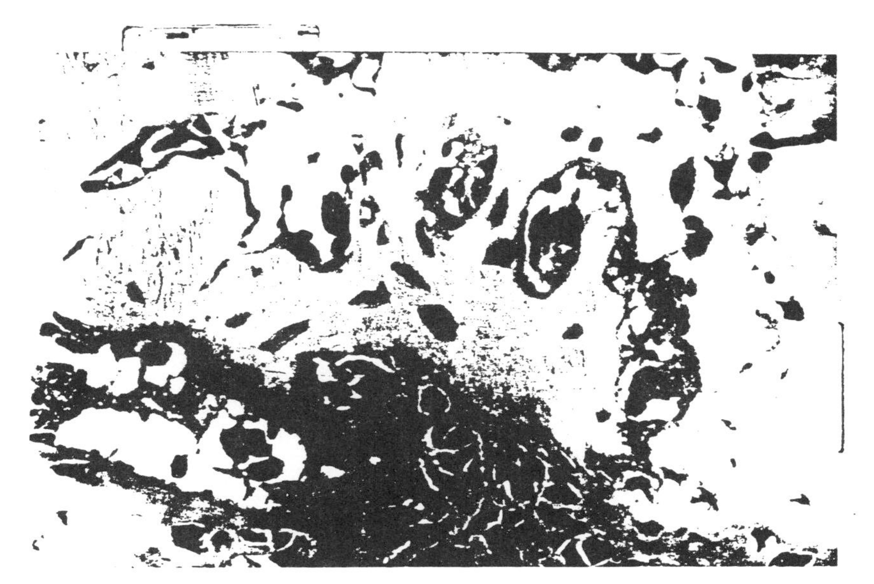

**FIGURE 12.3**
Delivery of BMP-3 from fibrin sealant. Purified bovine BMP-3 (100 $\mu$g/implant in 100 $\mu$L) was mixed with 25 mg of lyophilized insoluble collagenous bone matrix (ICBM) isolated from the long bones of rats and mixed with 60 $\mu$L of FS. The resulting clot was implanted, as described elsewhere in this volume [4], into the pectoralis major muscle of rats. The implants were harvested after twenty-eight days, sectioned, and stained with hematoxylin-eosin.

## DELIVERY OF FIBROBLAST GROWTH FACTORS FROM FIBRIN SEALANT

FS has also been shown to be an effective matrix for the delivery of various members of the FGF growth-factor family. In an experiment shown in Figure 12.4, FGF-1, along with a small concentration of heparin, was incorporated into FS that was placed into the lower well of a Boyden chemotaxis chamber. Human dermal fibroblasts were placed into the upper half of the chamber. In previous experiments it has been demonstrated that these cells, as well as the murine embryonic fibroblast cell line 3T3, exhibited a true chemotactic response to FGF-1, FGF-2, and FGF-4 [19]. In this experiment, the intent was to determine if inclusion of FGF-1 into, and release from, FS would alter this response. As shown in Figure 12.4, the fibroblasts migrated towards the FGF-1 containing FS in a dose-dependent fashion indicating that the FGF release from the FS retained this biological activity.

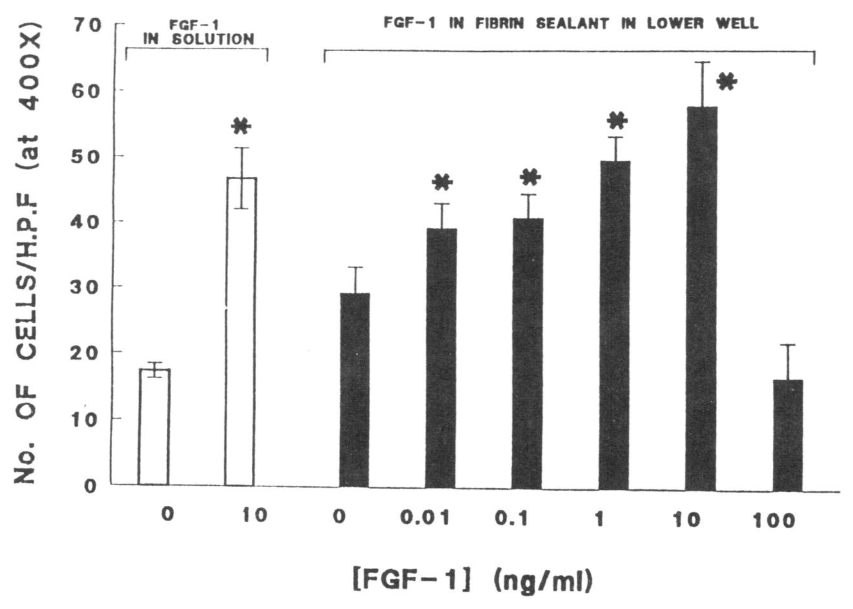


**FIGURE 12.4**
Migration of human dermal fibroblasts (HDF) toward FGF-1 released from fibrin sealant. FS containing different concentrations of FGF-1 and 10 units/mL of heparin was placed in the lower wells of modified Boyden's chemotaxis chambers divided by membranes with 12 $\mu$m pores. The upper and lower chambers were then filled with medium. Amounts of $5 \times 10^5$ HDF were placed in the upper chamber and the entire apparatus incubated for twelve hours at 37°C. The filters were then removed and fixed with glutaraldehyde and stained with Fisher's hematoxylin. The upper side of the filters were wiped off using a cotton swab. The filters were removed and mounted on microscope slides with their bottom side up. The filters were examined by microscopy. The results shown are the mean ± standard error of the number of migrated cells per high powered (400×) field from ten random fields from each of a set of triplicate chambers. Controls included the addition of medium alone or medium with 10 ng/mL of FGF-1, or FS alone, into the lower chamber (*: $p < 0.05$, Dunn's test).

Similar results were also found for FGF-2 and FGF-4 [19]. The decrease in cell migration at the highest concentration of FGF is a characteristic in vitro artifact of this type of migration assay. It is usually attributed to the rapid establishment of a concentration of chemoattractant that saturates the receptors of the responding cells while they are still in the upper chamber, thus preventing their directed migration.

The work of Greisler et al. [6] has shown that the lining of a porous vascular graft with FS supplemented with FGF-1 and heparin resulted in complete endothelialization of 23 cm-long grafts placed in dogs for one month. In this instance attraction and proliferation of endothelial cells and myofibroblasts by FGF-1 occurred in a predictable and directed fashion using FS as the delivery matrix. No signs of clotting, stenosis, or other undesirable responses were seen in the FS + FGF-1 treated grafts. Untreated grafts showed no endothelialization and the presence of multiple blood clots. After longer periods of implantation the FS was completely replaced with stable, well-vascularized tissue (H. Greisler, personal communication). Thus, the FS acted as an effective delivery vehicle for the growth factor by permitting the generation of desired new tissue that replaced the FS without undesirable side effects.

## DELIVERY OF TRIBUTYRIN FROM FIBRIN SEALANT

The induction of endothelialization of artificial vascular grafts by FGF-1 delivered in FS represents an important therapeutic application of the use of FS as a delivery vehicle. The exceptional biocompatibility of FS in exposure to the bloodstream [6] led to the investigation of additional vascular applications involving FS as a delivery vehicle for bioactive molecules. The treatment of localized vascular lesions, such as arteriosclerosis, is one such application. Excessive proliferation of smooth muscle cells in arterial walls is a significant component of this disease and in restenosis following angioplasty [21]. This led to the use of FS to deliver an antiproliferative or differentiating agent suitable for intravascular treatment. In choosing this agent it was thought important to use a drug with extremely low toxicity, as it was important not to induce cell damage that might exacerbate the underlying condition. Butyric acid has been shown to inhibit the proliferation of retinoblastoma cells [22], Swiss 3T3 cell [23], and other cell types [24] by inducing a differentiation program.

Work by G. Liau and N. Akhyani (unpublished data) has shown that these effects can also be induced in smooth muscle cells by the related compound, tributyrin. Unfortunately the desired effect requires a concentration of tributyrin that is close to saturation, making systemic therapy difficult. Therefore, a strategy of local therapy involving the delivery of tributyrin in FS directly to the lesion was pursued.

In a preliminary experiment to determine if this was feasible, tributyrin was mixed with thrombin, which was then mixed with fibrinogen to form FS. Culture medium was then placed in wells containing the FS-tributyrin, which were incubated at 37°C. The medium from a new set of three wells was harvested daily and the supernatant used to culture proliferating smooth muscle cells. After incubation for two days, the number of cells in each smooth muscle cell culture was measured using the MTS assay (similar to the MTT assay described earlier). As Figure 12.5 shows, the medium harvested from wells containing FS alone supported the growth of the smooth muscle cells, while the medium from wells with FS containing tributyrin significantly inhibited this proliferation. As the number of days increased of tributyrin diffusion into the medium, the degree of inhibition increased.

These results indicated that tributyrin can be delivered from FS for extended periods and that it retains the ability to inhibit the proliferation of smooth muscle cells. As a result of this successful demonstration of the ability of FS to serve as a delivery vehicle for tributyrin, experiments to further develop this system and to test it in vivo are currently under way.

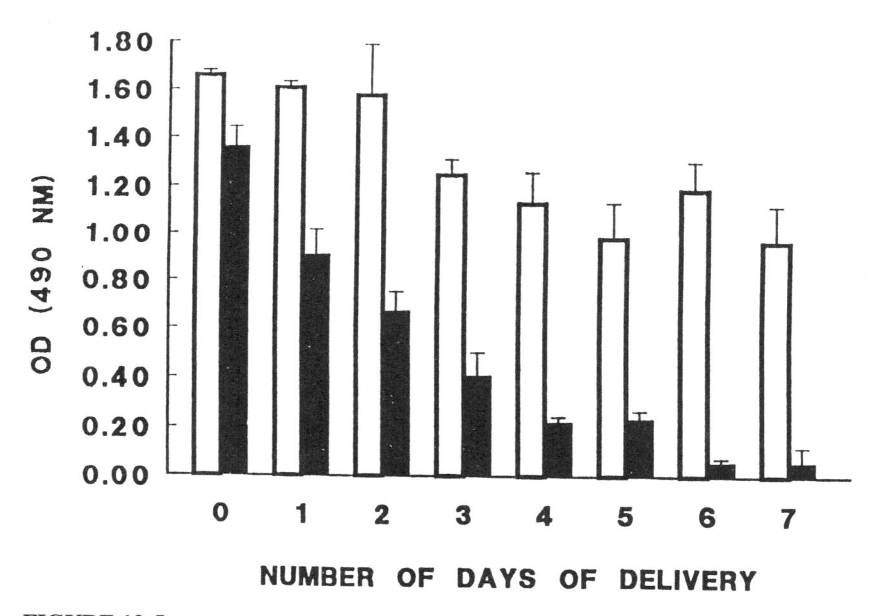


**FIGURE 12.5**
Inhibition of smooth muscle cell proliferation by tributyrin released from fibrin sealant. Tributyrin was incorporated into FS placed into twenty-four-well culture plates. Two milliliters of medium were added to each well and the plates incubated at 37°C. The medium from a new set of three wells was collected daily. These supernatants were then added to cultures containing 10,000 rat or rabbit smooth muscle cells per well that had been allowed to attach overnight. After a forty-eight hour incubation, the number of cells in each well was determined using the bioreduction of the tetrazolium compound MTS (Promega, Madison, WI) into a soluble formazan chromaphore detected by spectrophotometry at 490 nm (□: FS alone, ■: FS + tributyrin).

## CONCLUSIONS

Fibrin sealant has the characteristics of an excellent delivery vehicle for both drugs and biologics. It has been demonstrated that FS is capable of delivering chemotactic, growth promoting, and differentiation factors to induce both soft and hard tissue production or the inhibition of undesirable proliferation. It has also been used to deliver conventional pharmaceuticals in the form of antibiotics and chemotherapy drugs for prolonged periods. The diversity of compounds that can be delivered by FS, along with the compatibility of FS with living tissue and its well-established clinical safety record in Europe and Canada, indicate that it can be expected to play a significant role in future clinical applications of local delivery of drugs and biologics.

## REFERENCES

1. Mustoe, T., Pierce, G., Morishima, C., Deuel, T. Growth factor-induced acceleration of tissue repair through direct and inductive activities in a rabbit dermal ulcer model. *J. Clin. Invest.*, 87:694, 1991.
2. Matrix Pharmaceuticals, Inc. 1993. *F-D-C Reports—"The Pink Sheet"* T&G-15.
3. Saltz, R., Sierra, D., Feldman, D., Bartczak-Saltz, M., Dimick, A., Vasconez, L. O. Experimental and clinical applications of fibrin glue. *Plast. Reconstr. Surg.*, 88(6):1005, 1991.
4. Lasa, C., Hollinger, J., Drohan, W., MacPhee, M. Bone induction by demineralized bone powder and partially purified osteogenin using a fibrin-sealant carrier. In: *Surgical Adhesives and Sealants: Current Technology and Applications*. D. Sierra and R. Saltz, eds. Technomic Publishing Co., Inc., Lancaster, PA, 1996.
5. Kram, H., Bansal, M., Timberlake, O., Shoemaker, W. Antibacterial effects of fibrin glue-antibiotic mixtures. *J. Surg. Res.*, 50:175, 1991.
6. Greisler, H. P., Cziperle, D. J., Kim, D. U., Garfield, J. D., Petsikas, D., Murchan, P. M., Applegren, E. O., Burgess, W. H. Enhanced endothelialization of expanded polytetrafluoroethylene grafts by fibroblast growth factor type 1 pretreatment. *Surgery*, 112(2):244, 1992.
7. Greco, F., de Palma, L., Spagnolo, N., Rossi, A., Specchia, N., Gigante, A. Fibrin-antibiotic mixtures: An in vitro study assessing the possibility of using a biologic carrier for local drug delivery. *J. Biomed. Water. Res.*, 5:39, 1991.
8. Kovacs, B., Kerenyi, G. Bioplast® fibrin coagulum in large cystic defects of the jaw. *Int. J. Oral Surg.*, 5:111, 1976.
9. Goodson, J., HolBorow, D., Dunn, R., Hogan, P., Dunham, S. Monolithic tetracycline-containing fibers for controlled delivery to periodontal pockets. *J. Periodont.*, 544(10):575, 1983.
10. MacPhee, M., Nunez, H., Hennings, R., Campagna, A., Grummon, G., Harding, S., Drohan, W. Sustained release in vitro and in vivo of antibiotics from fibrin sealant. In: *Surgical Adhesives and Sealants: Current Technology and Applica-*

*tions,* D. Sierra and R. Saltz, eds. Technomic Publishing, Co., Inc., Lancaster, PA, 1996.

11. Yu, N., Palecek, J., Luck, E., Brown, D., Orenberg, E., Lalake, L., Shinn, J. Pharmacokinetics and clinical application of the intralesional methotrexate therapeutic implant. *Proceedings of ASCO 11,* March. Abs# 222:100. (Abstract), 1992.
12. Many innovative therapies for psoriasis hold promise. *Skin and Allergy News,* 22(10):1, 1991.
13. MacPhee, M., Campagna, A., Kidd, R., Best, A., Drohan, W. Fibrin sealant as a delivery vehicle for sustained and controlled release of chemotherapy agents. In: *Surgical Adhesives and Sealants: Current Technology and Applications,* D. Sierra and R. Saltz, eds. Technomic Publishing Co., Inc., Lancaster, PA, 1996.
14. Nicoletti, M., Lucchini, G., Massazza, G., Abbott, B., D'Incalci, M., Giavazzi, R. Antitumor activity of taxol (NSC-125973) in human ovarian carcinomas growing in the peritoneal cavity of nude mice. *Ann. Oncol.,* 4:151, 1993.
15. Markman, M., Rowinsky, E., Hakes, T., Reichman, B., Jones, W. Phase I trial of intraperitoneal taxol: A gynecologic oncology group study. *J. Clin. Oncol.,* 10(a):1485.
16. Rose, W. Taxol: A review of its preclinical in vivo antitumor activity. *Anti-Cancer Drugs,* 3:311, 1992.
17. Weiss, R., Donehower, D., Wiernik, D. Hypersensitivity reactions from taxol. *J. Clin. Oncol.,* 8:1263, 1990.
18. Arbuck, S., Canetta, R., Onetto, N., Christian, M. Current dosage and schedule issues in the development of paclitaxel (taxol). *Sem. Oncol.,* 20(4):31, 1993.
19. G-Nathan, S., MacPhee, M. Fibroblast chemotaxis towards fibroblast growth factors. *J. Cell. Biochem.,* S17E:120. (Abstract), 1993.
20. Weimar, B., Delvos, U. The mechanism of fibrin-induced disorganization of cultured human endothelial cell monolayers. *Arteriosclerosis,* 6:139, 1986.
21. Cercek, B., Sharifi, B., Barath, P., Bailey, L., Forrester, J. Growth factors in pathogenesis of coronary arterial restenosis. *Amer. J. Cardiol.,* 68:24C, 1991.
22. Kyritsis, A., Tsokos, M., Chander, G. Control of retinoblastoma cell growth by differentiating agents: Current work and future directions. *Anticancer Research,* 6:465, 1986.
23. Toscani, A., Soprano, D., Soprano, K. Sodium butyrate in combination with insulin or dexamethasone can terminally differentiate actively proliferating Swiss 3T3 cells into adipocytes. *J. Biol. Chem.,* 265(1):5722, 1990.
24. Prasad, K. Butyric acid: A small fatty acid with diverse biological functions. *Life Sciences,* 27:1351, 1980.

# *Chapter 13: Sustained Release of Antibiotics from Fibrin Sealant*

M. P. SINGH, R. BRADY, JR., W. DROHAN and M. J. MACPHEE

## INTRODUCTION

The administration of antibiotics is thought of as a commonplace matter. These drugs are usually given systemically in the hospital setting, and either systemically or topically under domestic circumstances. These approaches are generally adequate, largely due to the high therapeutic index of most antibiotics. Nevertheless, situations remain where the systemic administration of antibiotics produces unsatisfactory results.

Generally, this is due to either dose-limiting side effects or the inability of systemic administration to reach adequate tissue levels of the antibiotic. Severe trauma, such as large-area burns, may represent such a severe risk of infection that local delivery of high levels of antibiotics may be necessary. Chronic infections, such as periodontal disease, may require both high local levels of antibiotic and prolonged treatment. In both cases, achieving adequate local levels of antibiotics requires a delivery vehicle that is compatible with injured tissue, compatible with the processes of wound healing, and capable of delivering adequate quantities of antibiotic.

The use of fibrin sealant (FS) as a site-directed, drug-delivery system has potential for several clinical applications [1 – 3]. Unlike many nonbiological carriers and carriers derived from animal tissues, FS can be formulated to contain only human proteins, which minimizes immunogenicity and foreign body reactions. Fibrin is naturally present where tissue is damaged and, therefore, is at most sites where local antibiotic therapy is desirable. It can be expected not to interfere with the natural processes of healing and tissue remodeling.

Additionally, following drug delivery, physical removal of the FS from the recipient's tissue would not be required since it would be degraded by the host's natural fibrinolytic system. The degradation of FS is part of the body's natural processes of healing injured tissue; thus, it avoids the potential problems of excessive inflammation that may accompany artificial "biodegradable" delivery vehicles.

Several methods of delivering antibiotics to specific sites utilizing fibrin have been devised. Such "antibiotic-supplemented" fibrin has been shown to be useful in some clinical and preclinical settings. For example, it has been reported that antibiotic-supplemented fibrin sealant inhibits infections in vascular grafts [4], endocarditis [5], prosthetic heart valves [6], induced ossification of cystic defects of the jaw, and treatment of osteitis [7,8].

In these applications, two drawbacks of FS as a delivery system for antibiotics have been noted: the relatively small load of antibiotic that can be incorporated into the matrix and, more importantly, the relatively short duration of antibiotic release [8,9]. The short duration of release is due to fast rate of diffusion of small molecules by simple Fickian diffusion.

The studies presented in this report describe means to overcome these apparent deficiencies of FS as an antibiotic delivery system. The release rates can be retarded by using insoluble forms of antibiotics where the release mechanism is governed by a coupled diffusion-dissolution mechanism.

Drug release phenomena from monolithic matrices have generally been described by the solution of classical Fickian diffusion equation with appropriate boundary conditions. For the case of small molecules, such as antibiotics, the diffusion coefficient (D) is of the order of $40-60 \times 10^{-7}$ $cm^2/sec$ and the release rates are so fast that all the loaded antibiotic releases in a few hours.

One of the ways to retard the rate of release of the drug from such matrices is to provide a resistance other than diffusion in the release mechanism. By incorporating the drug above its solubility limit, it is possible to modulate the release rates by a coupled diffusion-dissolution mechanism.

For the case of a dissolution-controlled system, after an initial "burst" phase it is possible to obtain a long-term period of independent (i.e., linear or zero-order) release rates. In contrast, when the release is controlled by diffusion, the release rate will be proportional to the square root of time [10,11].

These theoretical analyses implied that dissolution of a solid drug would be a viable mechanism to control the drug release over an extended period of time in a controlled fashion. The feasibility of using this mechanism to obtain extended release of antibiotics from fibrin sealant was investigated for this chapter.

Tetracycline is an antibiotic with a broad spectrum of clinical uses. Additionally, it is easily quantified in solution by spectrophotometry. Tetracycline free-base has a very low solubility in aqueous media (0.4 mg/mL) [12].

Therefore, this investigation was conducted using tetracycline free-base as the antibiotic to be released.

The requirements for a suitable matrix to contain an antibiotic may vary depending upon the exact application; however, such a matrix will always need to be biodegradable in a physiological setting and through a pathway that does not alter or interfere with natural host defenses or healing. Additionally, it would seem likely that an adhesive matrix would also be desirable, as this would ensure that the matrix remained at the site of application. Fibrin sealant possesses these qualities.

Fibrin sealant is comprised of cross-linked fibrin units that are polymers of modified fibrinogen monomers. By altering the concentrations of fibrinogen in the fibrin-sealant matrix, it is possible to alter physical properties, such as the pore size of the cross-linked fibrin. This study reports the successful release of tetracycline from fibrin sealant for periods up to six weeks.

Also examined is the effect of fibrinogen concentration in the FS on the release kinetics of tetracycline. In addition, it can be demonstrated that by altering the concentration of the drug loaded it is possible to modulate the release rates.

## MATERIALS AND METHODS

### Fibrin Sealant

One hundred milligrams of freeze-dried human topical fibrinogen complex (TFC), which contained ¢85% fibrinogen as well as Factor XIII (American Red Cross, Rockville, MD), was mixed with 10 mg of freeze-dried human thrombin (American Red Cross, Rockville, MD) in the presence of 0.9 mL of 40 mM calcium chloride (American Reagent, Shirley, NY). To obtain lower concentrations of fibrinogen in the FS, the amount of TFC was decreased appropriately. Fibrinogen converted into cross-linked fibrin very rapidly and this was placed into a 20 mm × 10 mm × 3 mm mold and pressed to form a slab. Six-millimeter diameter disks were punched out by using a 6 mm biopsy punch (Acuderm Inc., Ft. Lauderdale, FL).

### Tetracycline-Supplemented Fibrin Sealant

To obtain tetracycline free-base (TET)-supplemented fibrin sealant (TET-FS), the desired amount of anhydrous TET (Sigma Chemical Co., St. Louis, MO) was hand mixed with TFC and thrombin. An appropriate amount of 40 mM $CaCl_2$ solution was added to form the clots as described above.

### Tetracycline Release in Vitro

The delivery of TET from TET-FS in vitro was investigated under two conditions. In the first, the "limited-sink" model, a small eluate volume was used with continuous eluate exchange at regular intervals without agitation. The TET-FS disks were placed into a well of a 24-well sterile tissue culture plate (Corning, Corning, NY). Phosphate-buffered saline (2 mL) was added to each well and subsequently collected and replaced daily. The supernatant samples were analyzed using spectrophotometry at 340 nm. Fibrin sealant disks containing no tetracycline were also investigated as controls.

The second condition utilized a large eluate volume (45 mL) and continuous agitation (the "infinite sink" model). The FS-TET disks were suspended in 45 mL of PBS in a 50 mL centrifuge tube that was inverted approximately twenty times per minute. The buffer was exchanged daily. All release experiments were performed at 37°C.

### Measurement of Tetracycline Concentrations

The concentrations of TET in the eluate samples from all the experiments were measured spectrophotometrically at a wavelength of 340 nm and calculated using a linear standard curve of tetracycline-HCL (Sigma, St. Louis, MO) covering concentrations from 0 to 200 $\mu$g/mL. When necessary, the samples were diluted with distilled water to be within the standard concentration range.

### Linear Regression

Linear regression analysis of cumulative mass deliveries was performed using commercial software (SlideWrite, Carlsbad, CA).

## RESULTS

### Kinetics of Release of TET from TET-FS

The tetracycline release results obtained under limited-sink conditions are shown in Figure 13.1. The concentration of the tetracycline in the eluent is plotted as a function of time. The TET-FS disks containing TET at a concentration of 340 mg/mL continued to release TET, as detected by

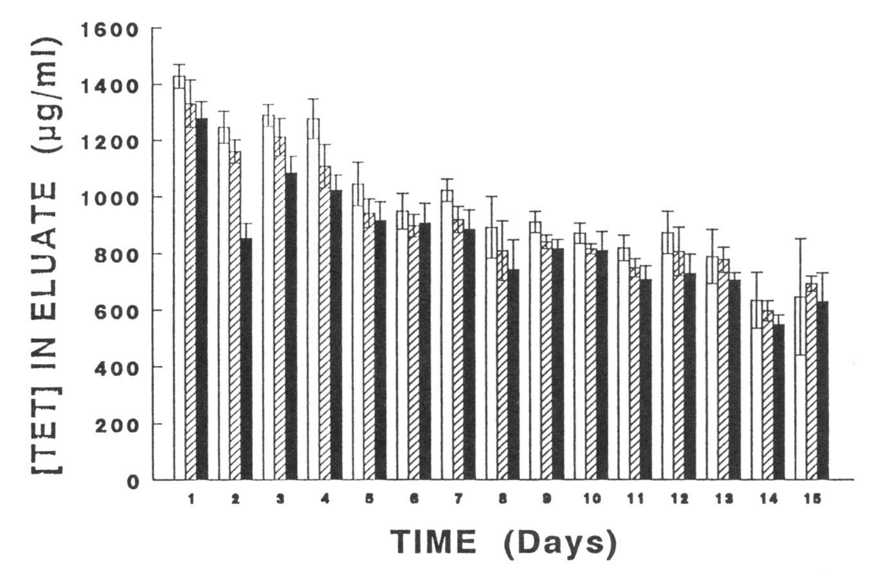


**FIGURE 13.1**
Release kinetics of TET from TET-supplemented fibrin sealant under limited-sink conditions in vitro. Fibrin-sealant disks (3 × 6 mm) containing 340 mg of tetracycline per mL of fibrin sealant containing 20 (□), 40 (▨), or 76 mg/mL (■) of fibrinogen were immersed in 2 mL of phosphate-buffered saline (PBS) at 37°C. The PBS was changed daily. The concentration of tetracycline in the PBS was measured by spectrophotometry at 340 nm.

spectrophotometry, for two weeks, while the eluate from control disks without TET produced no absorbance. The FS-TET disks delivered 1.3 mg/mL of eluate (equivalent to 2.6 mg/day) of tetracycline in twenty-four hours and the delivery rate remained above 2 mg/day for four days.

Thereafter, concentrations greater than 500 μg/mL were observed for another eleven days. While the delivery rates declined from day 1 to day 14, the decrease was very gradual. Even after fifteen days of release, less than 40% of the drug loaded had released indicating that release would continue for longer than two weeks. Figure 13.2 shows the cumulative release of tetracycline from the FS-TET matrices (with a fibrinogen concentration of 76 mg/mL) under limited-sink conditions as a function of time. As the figure shows, after four days a linear relationship existed between the amount released and the time period.

In order to determine the maximum possible release rate, TET release data were obtained using the infinite-sink model and are shown in Figure 13.3. While TET was released to a concentration of greater than 350 μg/mL

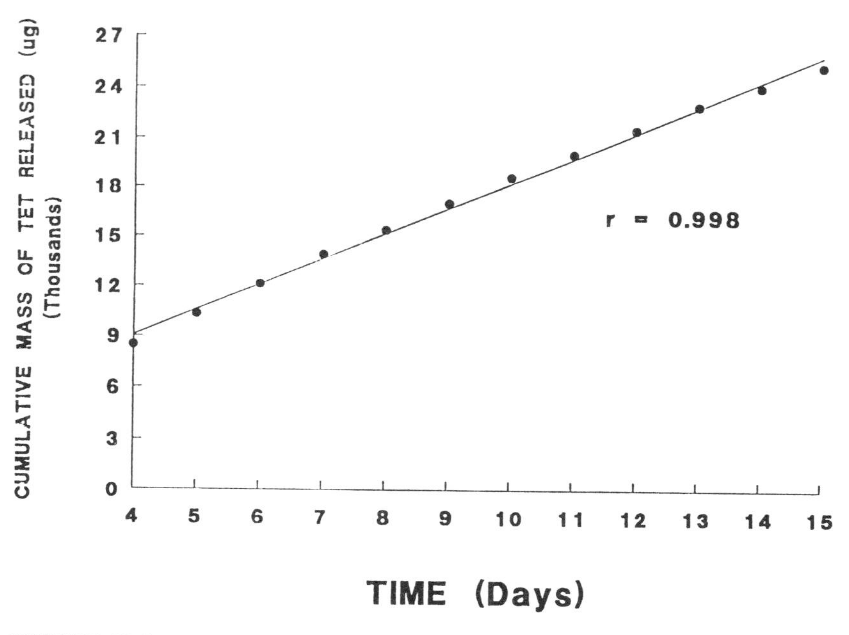


**FIGURE 13.2**
Cumulative release of TET as a function of time under limited-sink conditions (76 mg/mL of fibrinogen). The cumulative mass of TET released in the experiment shown in Figure 13.1 was calculated by adding the total amount released in the elution buffer until each time point.

during the first twenty-four hours, the concentration was maintained above 50 $\mu$g/mL for five days. The tetracycline concentration in the elution buffer remained above 5 $\mu$g/mL for an additional seven days. Controls containing no tetracycline were also analyzed and no absorbance was found at 340 nm indicating that neither the components nor any breakdown products of fibrin sealant interfered with the tetracycline analysis.

Figure 13.4 shows the cumulative release for the infinite-sink conditions as a function of square root of time. For prolonged periods after four days, a linear correlation between the amount released and square root of time was found.

Also investigated was the effect of fibrinogen concentration on the release kinetics of TET. Figure 13.1 shows the release of TET, under limited-sink conditions, from matrices containing fibrinogen at concentrations of 20 mg/mL, 40 mg/mL, and 76 mg/mL. For higher fibrinogen concentrations the release rates were slightly lower than at lower fibrinogen concentration. However, the differences are within the experimental error. Figure 13.3 shows the effect of fibrinogen concentration in the FS on the release kinetics of tetracycline under infinite-sink conditions. No relationship was observed

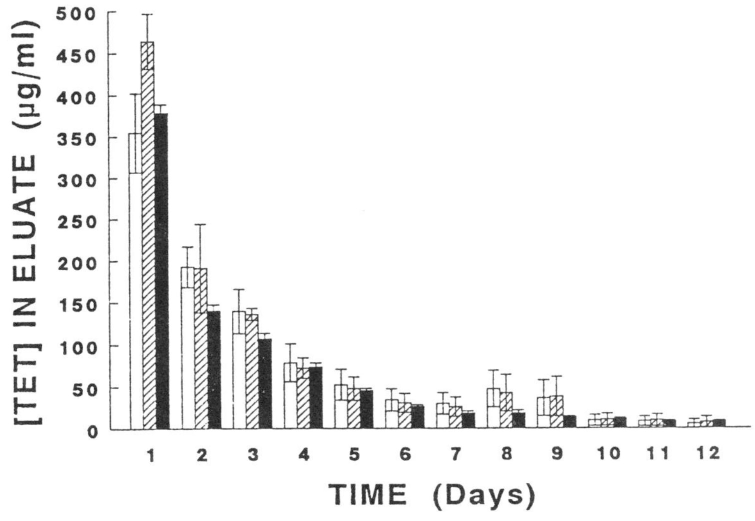


**FIGURE 13.3**
Release kinetics of TET from TET-supplemented fibrin sealant under infinite-sink conditions in vitro. Fibrin-sealant disks (3 × 6 mm) containing 340 mg of TET per mL of fibrin sealant containing 20 (□), 40 (▨), or 76 mg/mL (■) of fibrinogen were suspended in 45 mL of PBS at 37°C and vigorously stirred. The PBS was exchanged daily, and the concentration of tetracycline in the PBS measured spectrophotometry at 340 nm.

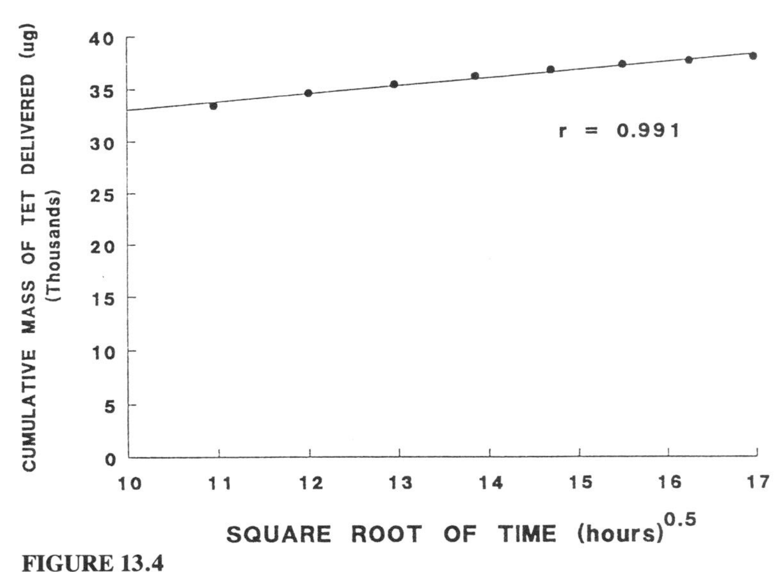


**FIGURE 13.4**
Cumulative release of TET from TET-supplemented fibrin sealant under infinite-sink conditions (76 mg/mL of fibrinogen). The cumulative mass of TET released in the experiment shown in Figure 13.3 was calculated by adding the total amount released in the elution buffer until each timepoint and is here plotted against the square root of time.

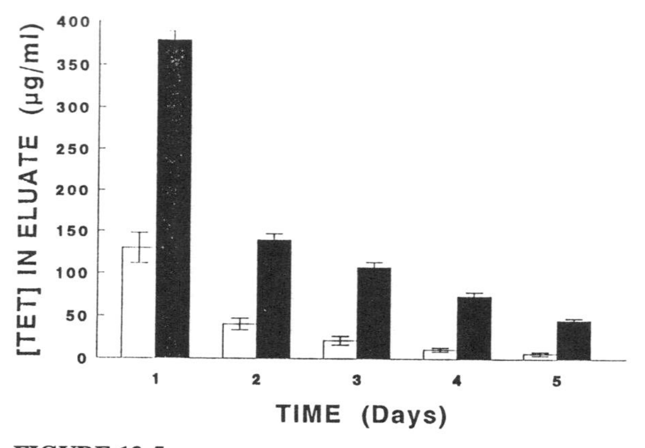


**FIGURE 13.5**
Effect of TET concentration loaded on the release kinetics from fibrin sealant. Fibrin-sealant disks (3 × 6 mm) containing either 345 (■) or 120 (□) mg of TET per mL of fibrin sealant were suspended in 45 mL of PBS at 37°C and vigorously stirred. The PBS was exchanged daily, and the concentration of tetracycline in the PBS measured by spectrophotometry at 340 nm.

between fibrinogen concentration and the release rate of TET under these conditions.

Figure 13.5 shows the effect of tetracycline concentration on the release kinetics from fibrin sealant under infinite-sink conditions. Lowering the tetracycline concentration loaded into the fibrin sealant resulted in a lower release rate. When 120 mg/mL of tetracycline were loaded, the initial burst was 130 μg/mL. This was three times lower than when 345 mg/mL of tetracycline were loaded.

## DISCUSSION

The objective of these studies was to develop a technique to deliver antibiotics using fibrin sealant as the delivery system for long periods in order to combat infection. In practical terms, it is necessary to include sufficient amounts of antibiotics into the fibrin matrix and deliver the antibiotics at an adequate concentration, rate, and duration. Previous attempts to accomplish this goal resulted in short delivery times, usually between one and five days (typically measured under limited-sink conditions), and often in low or inadequate concentration [4,5,8,13].

In contrast to these studies, which utilized antibiotic solutions to formulate the antibiotic-matrix, a highly insoluble form of the antibiotic was incorporated into the FS as a solid dispersed throughout the matrix. The delivery of the antibiotic, therefore, required both the dissolution of the solid into solution as well as the diffusion of the resulting ions through the FS matrix and into the surrounding environment. This resulted in a slow release of antibiotic from the matrix.

The use of an antibiotic in a chemical form with low solubility rendered the system susceptible to saturation-induced limitation of the delivery rate. When tested under limited-sink conditions, which tend to encourage such limitations, delivery times of over two weeks were attained in vitro. Under these conditions, a linear relationship between TET release and time was observed that indicates that the release is controlled by dissolution [10,11]. This indicates that the rate of dissolution was much smaller than the rate of diffusion; thus dissolution was the mechanism governing the release kinetics. After two weeks, less than half of the TET within the matrix had been released. As release was linearly related to time, it is possible to predict that a delivery duration in excess of one month would be expected from this system. This prediction has since been confirmed in a preliminary experiment (data not shown).

Under conditions in which the saturation effects were minimized and agitation was provided – infinite sink – it was expected that the rate of dissolution would be increased. Even under these extreme conditions it was possible to obtain delivery times of ten to twelve days. In this case the diffusion was the controlling mechanism, because dissolution is driven at a much higher rate. This is due to the mixing, agitation, and large eluate volume that results in a lower concentration of drug in solution within and immediately surrounding the matrix (boundary layers).

This resulted in a faster release rate compared to limited-sink condition and a linear relationship between the mass of drug released and the square root of time [10,11]. Under these most rigorous conditions, release of antibiotic continued for almost two weeks, and therapeutic concentrations ($\geq 50\ \mu g/mL$) were maintained in the 45 mL of eluate for five days. In terms of antibiotic concentration in the eluate, the use of a relatively insoluble solid form of the drug resulted in delivery under infinite-sink conditions that equals or surpassed that shown by previous investigators under limited-sink conditions [4,5,8,13].

While true infinite-sink modeling involves the continuous flow of fresh buffer over the delivery matrix in order to prevent limitation of the delivery rate by saturation of the buffer, in practice the techniques described here represented an adequate approximation of limiting conditions. Tetracycline concentrations in the eluate from "infinite-sink" conditions never approached those seen during the "limited-sink" experiments, indicating that the system was not undergoing significant saturation-based limitations on delivery rates.

This also demonstrates that the mechanism of release from these two systems is different. For the case of limited-sink conditions, dissolution is the controlling mechanism, while for the case of infinite-sink conditions it is diffusion that is controlling the rate of release. Both of these in vitro kinetics, occurring under their respective extreme conditions, resulted in deliveries that would likely be of use in clinical situations.

It remains to be seen which model of delivery most realistically represented the environment encountered in vivo in clinical conditions. It is possible that both models may be applicable, albeit to distinctly different situations. For example, in a vascular graft impregnated with drug-supplemented FS and exposed to a large blood flow, the release rate could be similar to the results from the infinite-sink experiment.

In contrast, a similar implant nestled in a dental pocket of a patient undergoing treatment for periodontitis where the flow of gingival crevicular fluid is only a few milliliters per day [9,14] might produce in vivo delivery kinetics similar to those observed in the limited-sink experiments in vitro. If this is the case, high local concentrations of TET for periods of weeks could be achieved using TET-FS to combat refractory local infections, for example, in periodontal diseases and osteomyelitis. In addition, under situations similar to the graft described above, antibiotic-supplemented FS may be used to inhibit bacterial colonization of biomedical implants or internal wound healing sites for up to ten to twelve days after surgery.

For most pathogens, an effective concentration of TET would be in the range of from 1 to 100 μg/mL [13,14–16]. For example, the organisms that are believed to be largely responsible for periodontal disease require from 8 to 64 μg/mL of TET to inhibit their growth [15]. Such levels were met or exceeded in vitro for fifteen and ten days in the limited-sink and infinite-sink experiments, respectively. These data indicate that under limited-sink conditions these concentrations would be met for at least a month. Thus, clinically relevant effects in vivo may also extend for a month or longer.

If this system were used to treat periodontal disease where the limited-sink conditions most realistically model the in vivo conditions, the tetracycline concentration that could be attained would be 100 times higher than the 4–8 μg/mL obtained with systemic administration. Additionally, this form of controlled local delivery of antibiotics would utilize small doses and consequently would be expected to have minimal side effects when compared to conventional modes of drug administration.

Preliminary evidence indicates that this may be the case. Early in vivo laboratory experiments have indicated that TET suspended in FS was significantly more effective at preventing mortality from peritonitis than TET alone (data not shown). The delivery of TET incorporated in FS permitted the administration of a large enough dose of antibiotic to produce a slow release resulting in levels of free antibiotic in the peritoneum sufficient to combat the infection for extended periods, while affording protection against what was an otherwise lethal dose of antibiotic. In effect, this resulted in a greater therapeutic index for the antibiotic when delivered in FS.

The different delivery kinetics seen in the infinite-sink versus limited-sink models represents possible performance profiles in different locations in vivo. It is obviously desirable to have additional ways of controlling the release profile. The nature of the microenvironment in which the matrices are implanted may not match the required release kinetics. Two possible methods for controlling the release kinetics from FS matrices were examined.

The first was to alter the concentration of fibrinogen used to form the delivery matrix. No substantial effect upon delivery was seen. The lowest concentration of fibrinogen gave essentially the same release kinetics as the higher concentrations, indicating that the pore size of FS was not sufficiently reduced by increasing the fibrinogen concentration to impede TET diffusion. At concentrations below 20 mg/mL the matrices did not have enough mechanical strength and were considered unviable for delivery purposes since the release rates would be altered by erosion or rupture of the matrix.

The second possible method to control the release profile was to alter the amount of TET loaded into the matrix. An examination of this possibility under infinite-sink conditions was made since sufficient levels and duration of delivery under limited-sink conditions had already been attained. Since a solid form of the antibiotic was used, loading of the FS with large amounts of antibiotic was easily accomplished. In practice, loadings of 345 mg/mL of matrix, in which the antibiotic represented 76% – 88% of the dry mass of the final matrix, were routinely accomplished. When these matrices were compared with ones with lower loadings of TET, both the initial burst concentration and the duration of delivery were greater when the amount of TET in the matrix was increased. Thus, the delivery duration may be controlled under infinite-sink conditions. Theoretically, duration of delivery under limited-sink conditions would also be related to the amount of TET loaded into the matrix. Preliminary experiments have been consistent with this prediction (data not shown).

The objective of this research is to develop a FS-based delivery vehicle for antibiotics and other therapeutically useful substances. Fibrin sealant has been shown to be an excellent carrier for demineralized bone matrix and its endogenous bone morphogenetic proteins to induce bone formation in otherwise nonhealing bone wounds in rats [2]. It may also serve as a carrier for antiproliferative compounds [1]. Greisler et al. have also used this fibrin sealant to deliver acidic, fibroblast growth Factor-1 to produce endothelialization of artificial vascular grafts in dogs [3]. Further characterization of the FS system is required to determine if clinically effective concentrations, release rates, and duration of protection can be obtained in order to combat infection in tissues. The results described here suggest that FS, adequately formulated, may be helpful as a biodegradable drug delivery vehicle for local antibiotic delivery in clinical situations.

## REFERENCES

1. MacPhee, M., Campagna, A., Kidd, R., Best, A., Drohan, W. Fibrin sealant as a delivery vehicle for sustained and controlled release of chemotherapy agents. In: *Surgical Adhesives and Sealants: Current Technology and Applications.* D. Sierra and R. Saltz, eds. Technomic Publishing Co., Inc., Lancaster, PA, 1996.
2. Lasa, C., Hollinger, J., Drohan, W., MacPhee, M. Bone induction by demineralized bone powder and partially purified osteogenin using a fibrin-sealant carrier. In: *Surgical Adhesives and Sealants: Current Technology and Applications.* D. Sierra and R. Saltz, eds. Technomic Publishing Co., Inc., Lancaster, PA, 1996.
3. Greisler, H. P., Cziperle, D. J., Kim, D. U., Garfield, J. D., Petsikas, D., Murchan, P. M., Applegren, E. O., Drohan, W., Burgess, W. H. Enhanced endothelialization of expanded polytetrafluoroethylene grafts by fibroblast growth factor type 1 pretreatment. *Surgery,* 112:244, 1992.
4. Sakurai, T., Nishikima, N., Yamamura, K., Shionoya, S. Controlled release of sisomicin from fibrin glue. *J. Cont. Rel.,* 18:39, 1992.
5. Deyerling, W., Haverich, A., Potel, J., Hetzer, R. A suspension of fibrin glue and antibiotic for local treatment of myocotic aneurysms in endocarditis—an experimental study. *Thorac. Cardiovasc. Surg.,* 32:369, 1984.
6. McGiffin, D. C., Galbraith, A., Wong, M., Burstow, D. Corynebacterium xerosis endocarditis of the aortic valve. Submitted for publication, 1995.
7. Kovacs, B., Kerenyi, G. Bioplast® fibrin coagulum in large cystic defects of the jaw. *Int. J. Oral Surg.,* 5:111, 1976.
8. Zilch, H., Lambiris, E. The sustained release of cefotaxim from a fibrin-cefotaxim compound in treatment of osteitis. *Arch. Ortho. Trauma Surg.,* 106:36, 1986.
9. Redl, H., Schlag, G., Stanek, G., Hirschl, A., Seelich, T. In vitro properties of mixtures of fibrin seal and antibiotics. *Biomaterials,* 4:29, 1983.
10. Harland, R., Dubernet, C., Benoit, J., Peppas, N. A model of dissolution-controlled, diffusional drug release from nonswellable polymeric microspheres. *J. Cont. Rel.,* 7:207, 1988.
11. Higuchi, T. Mechanism of sustained action medication. *J. Pharm. Sci.,* 52(12):1145, 1963.
12. Martindale. *The Extended Pharmacopeia.* J. Raynolds, ed. The Pharmaceutical Press, London, 1989.
13. Goodson, J., HolBorow, D., Dunn, R., Hogan, P., Dunham, S. Monolithic

tetracycline-containing fibers for controlled delivery to periodontal pockets. *J. Periodont.*, 54(10):575, 1983.

14. Goodson, J. Dental applications. In: *Medical Applications of Controlled Release. Vol. II., Applications and Evaluation.* R. S. Langer and D. L. Wise, eds. CRC Press, Inc., Boca Raton, Florida, p. 115, 1984.
15. Goodson, J., Offenbacher, S., Farr, D., Hogan, P. Periodontal disease treatment by local drug delivery. *J. Periodont.*, 56(5)265, 1985.
16. Goodson, J., Haffajee, A., Socransky, S. Periodontal therapy by local delivery of tetracycline. *J. Clin. Periodont.*, 6:83, 1979.

# *Chapter 14: Bone Induction by Demineralized Bone Powder and Partially Purified Osteogenin Using a Fibrin-Sealant Carrier*

C. LASA, JR., J. HOLLINGER, W. DROHAN and M. J. MACPHEE

## INTRODUCTION

A major challenge in the field of bone induction is the development of a suitable biocompatible and biodegradable carrier for bone morphogenetic proteins (BMPs). The carrier plays an important role in bone induction. It should place the BMPs at the desired location for bone deposition, prevent the prolapse of soft tissue into the skeletal defect, enable bone ingrowth, and maintain bony contours if necessary. The architecture of the vehicle must have an optimum mean pore size range, pore distribution, and pore volume that will support osteoconduction. Such a carrier must allow the sustained release of bone inductive proteins at the proper quantities and at appropriate times, and support the normal humoral and cellular activities involved in functional bone formation. It should also be completely absorbed so that it will not be an obstacle to bone repair [1].

A material that appears to meet many of the requirements for a delivery vehicle for BMPs is fibrin. Fibrin is an organic, biodegradable material derived from human plasma. Clinically, fibrin is nonantigenic and has angiotropic, hemostatic, and osteoconductive properties [2].

Commercial fibrin sealant from pooled, virally-inactivated human plasma has been used clinically as a hemostatic agent in Europe and Canada [3]. It is made by mixing concentrated fibrinogen and thrombin solutions to simulate the final stages of the normal coagulation cascade to form a clot. It is degraded by enzymatic fibrinolysis and phagocytosis. This study investigates the use of fibrin sealant as a carrier for known osteoinductive substances, such as demineralized bone and osteogenin.

## MATERIALS AND METHODS

### Fibrin Sealant (FS)

Concentrated fibrinogen complex was produced from fresh-frozen, pooled human plasma for the American Red Cross, Rockville, MD. The manufacturing process includes solvent/detergent treatment which inactivates lipid (and some nonlipid)-enveloped viruses [4]. The product was supplied in lyophilized form and reconstituted with sterile water. Mixing with 3.3 mL of sterile water resulted in a fibrinogen solution with the following characteristics: total protein, 120 mg/mL; fibrinogen, 90 mg/mL; fibronectin, 13.5 mg/mL; Factor XIII, 17 units/mL; and plasminogen, 2.2 $\mu$g/mL. The total protein concentration of the fibrinogen solution was varied depending on the total amount of sterile water used for reconstitution. In this study, fibrinogen solutions, with 10, 20, 30, 40, 60, 80, and 120 mg/mL total protein concentrations were used.

Concentrated thrombin was also produced from fresh-frozen, pooled human plasma. Its manufacturing process also included a solvent/detergent treatment step. The thrombin product was supplied in lyophilized form, reconstituted, and serially diluted with 40 mM calcium chloride solution to a concentration of 15 units/mL. Equal volumes of fibrinogen and thrombin solutions were mixed to produce fibrin sealant.

### Implant Preparation; DBP Study

(1) DBP + FS. Rat demineralized bone powder (DBP) was prepared as previously described [5]. Twenty-five milligrams of rat DBP (75 – 200 $\mu$ particle size) were added into a cylindrical aluminum mold chamber. Thirty microliters of fibrinogen solution was then pipetted onto the DBP and mixed thoroughly. Thirty microliters of thrombin solution (15 units/mL) were then added to the DBP-fibrinogen complex, mixed, and compressed to form a disk. The final concentrations of the fibrin sealant after mixing with DBP were 4, 8, 15, and 45 mg/mL (total protein). Disk-shaped implants 1 mm thick and 8 mm in diameter were formed.

(2) DBP alone. Disk implants composed of 25 mg DBP/implant were made.

(3) FS alone. Disk implants composed of fibrin sealant alone (using 4 and 45 mg/mL concentration) were likewise made using the same mold.

| Distribution of Implants | $n$[1] |
|---|---|
| DBP alone | 12 |
| DBP + FS (4 mg/mL) | 11 |
| DBP + FS (8 mg/mL) | 11 |
| DBP + FS (15 mg/mL) | 11 |
| DBP + FS (45 mg/mL) | 10 |
| FS alone, 4 mg/mL | 13 |
| FS alone, 45 mg/mL | 12 |

Implants were then placed in sterile nylon bags (measuring 1 cm × 1 cm) with a mesh size of 70 microns.

In a separate group of animals, DBP-FS implants were made in different shapes: triangles, squares, and doughnuts. Fifty milligrams of DBP were poured into the aluminum mold, to which 60 μL each of fibrinogen and thrombin solutions were added and mixed thoroughly. A disk-shaped implant with a diameter of 10 mm and a thickness of 2 mm was produced. The disk was then cut and trimmed manually into the desired shape.

There were four each of the square-, triangle-, and doughnut-shaped implants.

## Implant Preparation; Osteogenin Study

(1) Osteogenin-ICBM. Partially purified osteogenin was prepared as previously described [6]. Each implant consisted of 100 μL of osteogenin solution (1 mg/mL concentration) reconstituted with 25 mg of insoluble collagenous bone matrix (ICBM).
(2) Osteogenin-ICBM + FS. Another treatment arm consisted of osteogenin-ICBM implants (prepared as described above) to which 30 μL of fibrinogen solution and 30 μL of thrombin solution (0.01 units/mL) were added to produce FS concentrations of 15 and 30 mg/mL.
(3) ICBM alone. Implants consisting of insoluble collagenous bone matrix alone were made (as described above for osteogenin-ICBM) to serve as negative controls.

In a separate group of animals, osteogenin solution alone (1 mg/mL concentration, 100 μL aliquots) was mixed with 30 μL fibrinogen solution and 30 μL thrombin solution (0.01 units/mL) to evaluate whether osteogenin

[1] $n$: Number of implants used in this study.

| Distribution of Implants | $n$[1] |
|---|---|
| Osteogenin + ICBM | 16 |
| Osteogenin + ICBM + FS 15 mg/mL | 14 |
| Osteogenin + ICBM + FS 30 mg/mL | 15 |
| ICBM alone | 17 |

would still induce bone formation without its reconstitution with ICBM. There were 14 osteogenin-ICBM implants (positive controls), 12 ICBM implants (negative controls), 15 implants made of osteogenin + FS 15 mg/mL, and 15 implants made of osteogenin + FS 30 mg/mL.

## Animals

Male Long-Evans rats were obtained from Charles River Laboratories (Wilmington, MA). Animals were housed in separate cages after surgery in an animal care facility. Regular animal care and monitoring were provided by professionals who followed N.I.H. guidelines. All procedures performed were approved by the Animal Care and Use Committee of the Holland Laboratory.

## Surgery

Animals were anesthetized with a mixture consisting of 10 mL ketamine hydrochloride (Vetalar®, 100 mg/mL, Parke-Davis, Morris Plains, NJ), 5 mL xylazine (Rompun®, 20 mg/mL, Mobay Corporation, Shawnee, KS), and 1 mL physiological saline (0.9% NaC1), at a dose of 0.14 mL per 100 grams body weight, administered intramuscularly. After the anesthesia had taken effect, the operative site was prepped with 70% alcohol solution. The surgical procedure was then performed using aseptic technique.

A midline ventral incision was made and a space was created under the pectoralis major muscle using blunt dissection. A nylon envelope containing the designated experimental material was inserted into the space and secured with a 3-0 Dexon suture. This was repeated at the contralateral side. The skin was then closed with staples.

## Retrieval of Implants

Implants were retrieved four weeks postoperatively. Following euthanasia of the animals, a skin incision was made around the recipient bed

[1]$n$: Number of implants used in this study.

and soft tissues were reflected. Sharp and blunt dissection was used to recover the implants.

### Radiography

Implants were radiographed using the X-OMATL high contrast Kodak X-ray film (Eastman Kodak Company, Rochester, NY), in a Minishot Benchtop Cabinet X-ray System (TFI Corporation, West Haven, CT) at 30 Kvp, 3 mA for ten seconds. Gray-level densities of radiographs were analyzed using a Cambridge 920 Image Analysis System (Cambridge Instruments Limited, Cambridge, England).

### Radiomorphometry

X-rays of the implants were obtained at necropsy. Radiographs were projected onto a computer screen and the gray-scale processing capabilities of the computer used to compare the implant with a previously calibrated standard to derive radio-opacity values.

### Statistical Analysis

The InStat® statistical software package (GraphPad Software, San Diego, CA) was used for analysis of variance and Dunn's multiple-comparisons post-tests to determine differences between treatment groups.

### Histological Analysis

Specimens were placed immediately into labeled containers with 10% buffered formalin solution and submitted to a histology laboratory for processing.

## RESULTS

There were no significant differences in radio-opacity measurements between DBP disks and DBP + FS disks. There were also no significant differences within the DBP + FS group using different FS concentrations. However, when compared to FS implants, DBP and DBP + FS percent opacity values were significantly different from percent opacity values ($p < 0.01$), except for DBP + FS4 versus FS45 and DBP + FS45 versus FS4 and FS45. Although the difference was not statistically significant for these latter groups, the radio-opacity values were much higher for the DBP + FS groups than for the FS groups (Figure 14.1). Radio-opacity values were later correlated with histological findings.

DBP-FS implants in the form of squares, triangles, or doughnuts displayed radio-opaque images. The original shapes of the implants were generally retained. Radiomorphometry was not done for this small group of implants.

There were no significant differences between implants containing osteogenin (Figure 14.2). However, radio-opacity values of osteogenin-containing implants were significantly different from ICBM implants, ($p < 0.0001$). Radio-opacity values were later correlated with histologic findings.

In the other set of animals where evaluation of the osteoinductive property of osteogenin was evaluated without use of a collagen matrix, no radiomorphometry was done. Implants were examined histologically.

## Histology of Implants

At twenty-eight days postimplantation, most of the demineralized bone

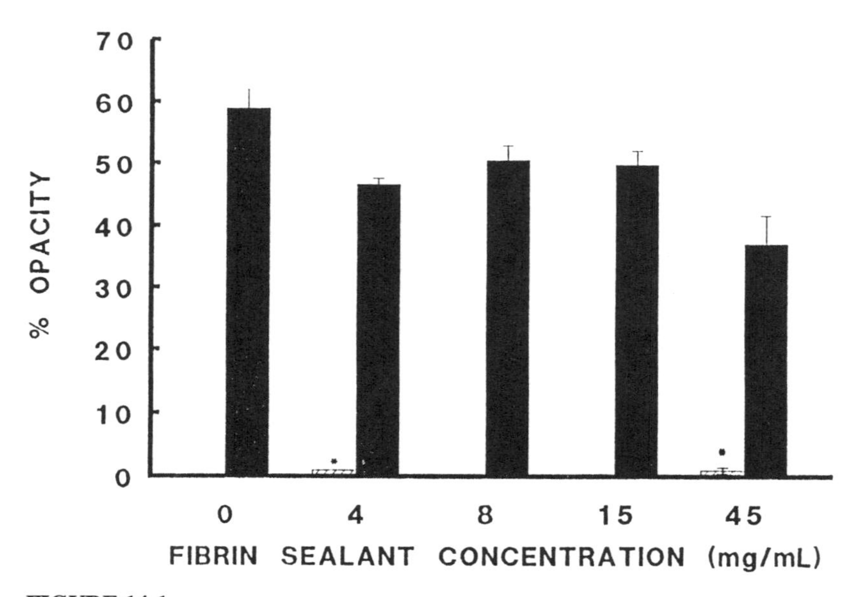


**FIGURE 14.1**
Radio-opacity values of DBP/FS implants. The black bars represent percent opacity values derived from DBP implants combined with different fibrinogen concentrations. Striped bars depict percent opacity values of fibrin implants alone. (*:Near-zero values are exaggerated to make them visible.)

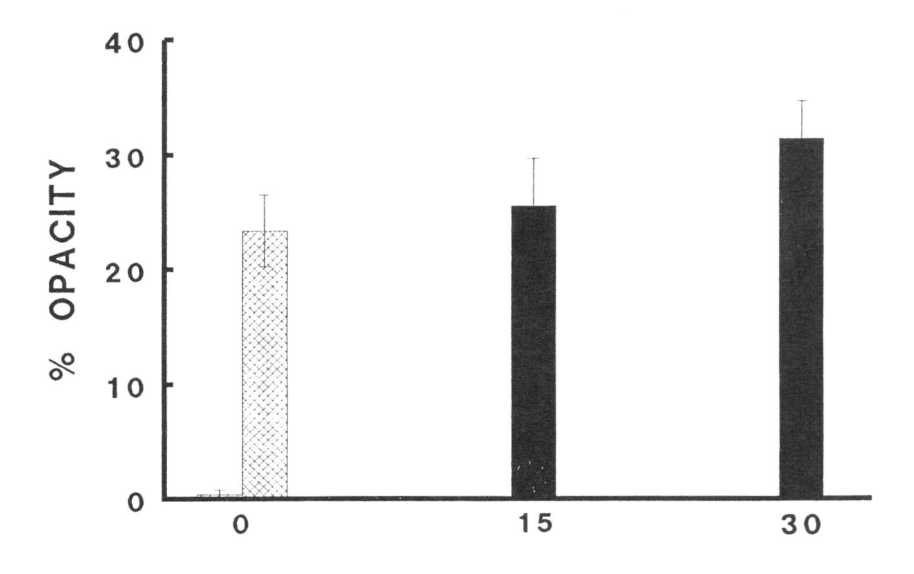


**FIGURE 14.2**
Radio-opacity values of osteogenin/ICBM implants. The black bars represent percent opacity values derived from osteogenin + ICBM implants combined with different fibrinogen concentrations. The hatched bar depicts osteogenin + ICBM alone, and the striped bar depicts ICBM alone.

particles that were either implanted alone or in a fibrin sealant matrix showed trabecular bone formation. Intertrabecular spaces were filled with bone marrow elements. High-power magnification clearly showed the presence of osteoblasts adjacent to newly deposited osteoid matrix. In areas where bone had been deposited, osteocytes were present within lacunar spaces. DBP + FS implants showed more cellularity, denser connective tissue, and greater neovascularization than DBP alone. No visible fibrin sealant matrix was evident within the ossicle. There was no evidence of a marked inflammatory response to the implant.

Histology of osteogenin + ICBM + FS implants showed new trabecular bone formation with intertrabecular myeloid elements, comparable to osteogenin + ICBM controls.

Osteogenin + FS implants likewise showed good ossicle formation and bone-marrow formation. The size of the ossicle corresponded with the original size of the whitish precipitate that was implanted. There were no obvious histological differences between the different concentrations of FS used as carriers for osteogenin. The original fibrin-sealant matrix was not discernible within the new trabecular bone that formed.

Radio-opacity values were correlated with histologic findings. These values corresponded with immature woven bone in the implants examined.

## DISCUSSION

The use of fibrin sealant as a delivery system for bone inductive proteins has been reported by previous investigators. Schwartz et al. implanted allogeneic DBP and bone matrix gelatin with or without fibrin sealant in heterotopic and orthotopic sites in rats [7]. They were not able to demonstrate a positive or negative effect of FS on bone induction. However, they noted that FS facilitated application of smaller particles of bone-matrix gelatin and prevented hematoma formation.

Kawamura and Urist used FS to deliver partially purified bone morphogenetic protein and reported a synergistic effect [2]. They speculated that fibrin sealant stopped bleeding, leading to a BMP concentration gradient that optimized cell to protein interaction leading to new bone formation.

These studies demonstrated that FS did not inhibit or delay the process of bone induction. As a carrier for demineralized bone particles, it improved the physical handling of DBP and allowed it to be molded into a desired shape. Absence of a marked inflammatory response to the implants in a FS matrix is an indication of its biocompatible property.

As a carrier for osteogenin reconstituted with ICBM, FS supported new bone formation. When osteogenin + ICBM implants were mixed with FS, the radiomorphometry measurements were not significantly different compared to osteogenin + ICBM alone. For osteogenin alone, studies demonstrated that new bone can be formed using a FS carrier in the absence of a collagen matrix. This is contrary to a previous suggestion that both the partially purified osteogenin and a species-specific collagenous bone matrix are required for bone induction [8]. The amount of bone that can be formed is, however, limited to the amount of osteogenin solution that can be contained within the fibrin matrices. At twenty-eight days postimplantation, the fibrin-sealant matrix was noted to have been completely resorbed in most of the implants in which it was used as a carrier.

## CONCLUSION

Fibrin sealant appears to possess an appropriate microarchitecture, biodegradation profile, and release kinetics to support osteoinduction by demineralized bone powder and partially purified osteogenin. Fibrin sealant also imparts desirable handling characteristics to the osteoinductive implants. Most significantly, it permits the induction of bone of a desired shape. Further studies should be undertaken to determine whether FS may be a suitable carrier for the highly purified recombinant bone morphogenetic proteins.

## REFERENCES

1. Hollinger, J. Factors for osseus repair and delivery. *J. Craniofacial Surg.*, 4:135–141, 1993.
2. Kawamura, M., Urist, M. R. Human fibrin is a physiological delivery system for bone morphogenetic protein. *Clin. Ortho. Rel. Res.*, 235:302–310, 1988.
3. Gibble, J. Ness, P. Fibrin glue: The perfect operative sealant? *Transfusion,* 30:741, 1990.
4. Fricke, W., Lamb, M. Viral safety of clotting factor concentrates. *Sem. Thromb. Hemostas.*, 19:56, 1993.
5. Mark, D., Hollinger, J. Hastings, C., et. al. Repair of calvarial nonunions by osteogenin, a bone-inductive protein. *Plast. Reconstr. Surg.*, 86:624, 1990.
6. Sampath, T., Muthukumaran, N., Reddi, A. H. Isolation of osteogenin, an extracellular matrix-associated, bone-inductive protein, by heparin affinity chromatography. *Proc. Natl. Acad. Sci. USA,* 84:7109, 1987.
7. Schwarz, N., Reddi, H., Schlag, G., et al. The influence of fibrin sealant on demineralized bone matrix-dependent osteoinduction. *Clin. Ortho. Rel. Res.*, 238:282–287, 1989.
8. Muthukumaran, N., Ma, S., Reddi, A. H. Dose-dependence of and threshold for optimal bone induction by collagenous bone matrix and osteogenin-enriched fraction. *Coll. Relat. Res.*, 8:433, 1988.

# *Chapter 15: Fibrin Sealant as a Delivery Vehicle for Sustained and Controlled Release of Chemotherapy Agents*

M. J. MACPHEE, A. CAMPAGNA, A. BEST, R. KIDD and W. DROHAN

## INTRODUCTION

The treatment of neoplastic disease represents a major challenge to modern medicine. When a well-defined tumor is evident and accessible, surgical resection is the usual first step. In recent years, subsequent, or "adjuvant," therapy has gained increasing acceptance as the second step in cancer treatment. Adjuvant therapy may involve radiation, antiproliferative drugs, hormone analog treatment, or immunotherapy. Of these, radiation and antiproliferative compounds currently represent the most common therapy.

Both antiproliferative drugs and radiation target proliferating cells regardless of whether they are malignant or normal. Since there are numerous tissues in which cellular proliferation is a normal and necessary activity, systemic treatment is likely to affect these tissues, resulting in undesirable side effects. In order to minimize these effects, radiation treatment is only used to treat relatively small volumes of tissue. Unfortunately, the selective administration of chemotherapy drugs is not as easily accomplished, and the majority of hemotherapies are administered systemically. In systemic chemotherapy, the antiproliferative drug is distributed throughout the body in a fairly even manner. As a result, proliferating cells in healthy organs are exposed to nearly the same concentration of drugs as those in tumors. Indeed, several factors in the hemodynamics of tumors may actually prevent an even distribution of drugs into tumors, further aggravating the problem [1–3].

The desirable effects of most chemotherapy agents depend upon the differences in the proliferation rates between those normal cells that proliferate and the cancer cells that are the target of treatment. Since these rates may be similar, the results are unpleasant side effects that are usually dose-limiting. It is generally believed that the higher the concentration of chemotherapy the tumor can be exposed to and the longer the duration of exposure, the greater the efficacy of the treatment. The effectiveness of most antiproliferative chemotherapy is limited by the severity of these side effects.

One approach to circumvent this problem is the local or regional treatment of tumors with chemotherapy drugs. This involves introducing the drugs into or onto the tumor itself (local) or into a body cavity in which the tumor resides (regional), such as the peritoneum or cerebral vesicles. Both of these approaches serve to generate a concentration gradient in which the highest drug concentrations are maintained in and/or around the tumor. The result is that for a given concentration of drug within the tumor, not only is the concentration in other tissues markedly less, there is also the expectation of less severe side effects.

Local delivery of chemotherapeutics requires a suitable drug-delivery vehicle. Several approaches have been tried, and the most successful to date has been a protein matrix [4–10]. While clinical trials with this vehicle have been successful, an even more suitable vehicle may be human fibrinogen [10]. When combined with thrombin and Factor XIII, fibrinogen is converted to fibrin and is covalently bound to the surrounding proteins. The result is a hemostatic adhesive, which will be naturally broken down by the body. Such a delivery vehicle would have the highly desirable characteristics of preventing bleeding from the administration site(s) as well as remaining precisely where it was implanted owing to its natural adhesion to existing protein structures [11,12].

If fibrinogen is to be used as a delivery vehicle for chemotherapeutics, it will have to permit the loading of adequate quantities of drugs, which must be released in sufficient concentration to kill the surrounding tumor cells and for a long enough period to diffuse throughout the tumor mass. Fibrin sealant (FS), a gel similar to a natural clot, is formed by mixing concentrates of virally-inactivated human fibrinogen and thrombin solutions. It has been used mostly as a hemostatic and/or adhesive agent in Europe and Canada for over a decade.

The possible use of FS as a delivery vehicle for the chemotherapy agent 5-fluorouracil (5-FU) has been explored. Murine renal cell carcinoma cell line RENCA as target cells were used since this is a spontaneously arisen Balb/c neoplasm that lends itself to research in vivo [13]. Results demonstrate that human fibrin can indeed serve to deliver 5-FU in concentrations sufficient to kill tumor cells. When the anhydrous form of 5-FU is used, delivery can be extended up to 120 hours.

## MATERIALS AND METHODS

### Reagents

Fibrin sealant was obtained from the American Red Cross (Rockville, MD). Both the topical fibrinogen complex (TFC), which contained fibrinogen and Factor XIII and the thrombin component, were produced from fresh-frozen, pooled human plasma that was virally inactivated by using the solvent detergent method [14]. Both the TFC and thrombin were provided in lyophilized form. Each vial of TFC was reconstituted with 3.3 mL of sterile water and diluted 1:1 with histidine buffer. This resulted in a solution with the following component: total protein, 60 mg/mL; fibrinogen, 45 mg/mL; fibronectin, 6.75 mg/mL; Factor XIII, 8.5 units/mL; and plasminogen, 1.1 μg/mL. Concentrated thrombin was reconstituted and diluted with 40 mM calcium chloride solution to a concentration of 15 units/mL. Equal volumes of fibrinogen and thrombin solutions were mixed to produce the fibrin sealant. The agent 5-FU was obtained from Sigma (St. Louis, MO). Phosphate buffered saline (PBS) was obtained from Gibco (Grand Island, NY). Histidine buffer consisted of 0.05M histidine + 0.15M NaCl, pH 7.3.

### Preparation of FS + 5-FU Clots

Fibrin sealant, with or without 5-FU, was formed by mixing equal volumes of TFC and thrombin solutions in the presence or absence of 5-FU. When 5-FU was included in the liquid form, a saturated solution (15 mg/mL) was prepared in histidine buffer or 40 mM $CaCl_2$. These solutions were then used to reconstitute the lyophilized components of the fibrin sealant as described above. When the 5-FU was in the anhydrous state, it was mixed with the FS and the fibrin allowed to gel. The final volume of the clots was 400 μL.

### Determination of 5-FU Release Kinetics

The 5-FU-FS mixtures were placed into 2 mL of PBS, which was changed daily (limited-sink conditions (LS)), or into 45 mL of PBS, which was continuously agitated and sampled at various intervals (infinite-sink conditions (IS)). All experiments were carried out at 37°C. Concentrations of 5-FU in the eluates were measured spectrophotometrically at 260 μm.

### Statistics

Linear regressions and regression coefficients were performed using commercial software (SlideWrite® Plus, Advanced Graphics Software Inc., Carlsbad, CA).

## RESULTS

### Duration of Delivery of 5-FU from FS Is Extended by the Use of the Anhydrous Form

Initial experiments suggested that the duration of delivery of 5-FU from the FS clots was limited to approximately six hours (data not shown). In order to increase this, 5-FU was loaded into the clots in anhydrous form. When a saturated solution of 5-FU was employed to reconstitute both the TFC and thrombin, the total amount of 5-FU in the FS clots was 7 mg. Accordingly, 7 mg of anhydrous 5-FU was formulated into a second group of clots. It was found that substantially more than 7 mg of anhydrous 5-FU could be loaded into the clots, so another group with 50 mg of anhydrous 5-FU/clot was also made. When these clots were tested under limited-sink conditions, both the soluble and anhydrous 5-FU at 7 mg/clot delivered the majority of their material in six hours (Figure 15.1). In contrast, the clots loaded with 50 mg of 5-FU delivered their contents for twenty-four hours before delivery began to drop off, with delivery lasting for between fifty to eighty hours.

### Duration of Delivery of 5-FU from FS Is Proportional to the Mass of Anhydrous 5-FU

Since the duration of delivery of 5-FU was increased when the mass of anhydrous 5-FU was increased, the maximum duration of delivery attainable was sought by increasing the amount of 5-FU in the FS. It was found that 200 mg of 5-FU was the maximum that could be loaded into the 400 $\mu$L clots. The results in Figure 15.2 show that when these clots were tested under limited-sink conditions, delivery was maintained for four hours when 7 mg of soluble or anhydrous 5-FU was loaded into the clots; for thirty hours with 50 mg; and for eighty-three hours with 200 mg of anhydrous 5-FU.

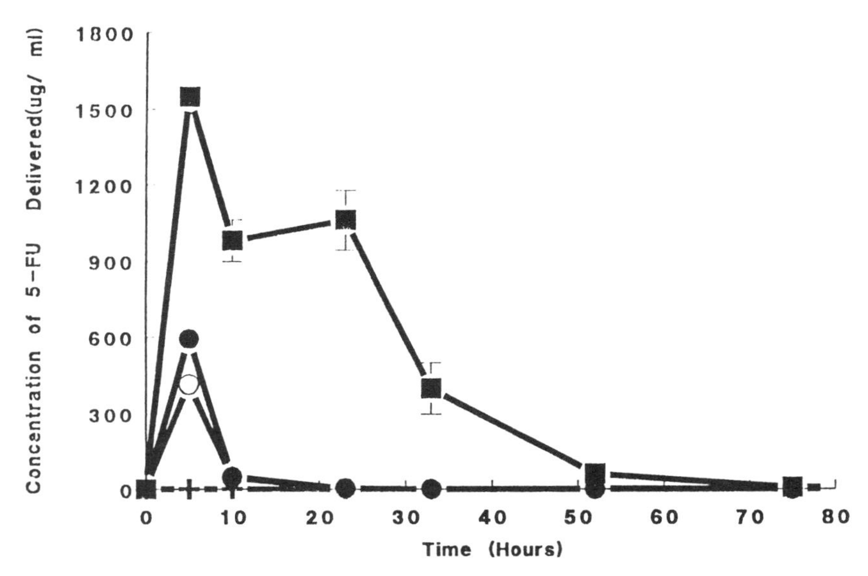


**FIGURE 15.1**
Concentration of 5-FU delivered from fibrin sealant clots under limited-sink conditions. Fibrin sealant clots with a volume of 400 $\mu$L and containing various amounts of 5-FU were placed in 2 mL of buffer that was exchanged every twenty-four hours. The concentration of 5-FU released into the eluate was determined spectrophotometrically. (+): FS alone, (O): FS with 7 mg of aqueous 5-FU, (¢ ): FS with 7 mg of anhydrous 5-FU, ($_6$ ): FS with 50 mg of anhydrous 5-FU.

## The Rate of Delivery of 5-FU from FS Is Constant under Limited-Sink Conditions

The data in Figure 15.2 also indicated that the rate of delivery was proportional to the mass of 5-FU in each clot and that these rates remained constant for each group.

## The Rate of Delivery of 5-FU from FS Is Constant under Infinite-Sink Conditions

In order to maximize the delivery rate, the eluate size was increased in order to exceed the volume required to dissolve all the 5-FU in the clots. The system was agitated constantly. Under these "infinite-sink" conditions the delivery rates for clots containing 50 or 200 mg of anhydrous 5-FU were determined. Delivery rates were found to be constant and delivery con-

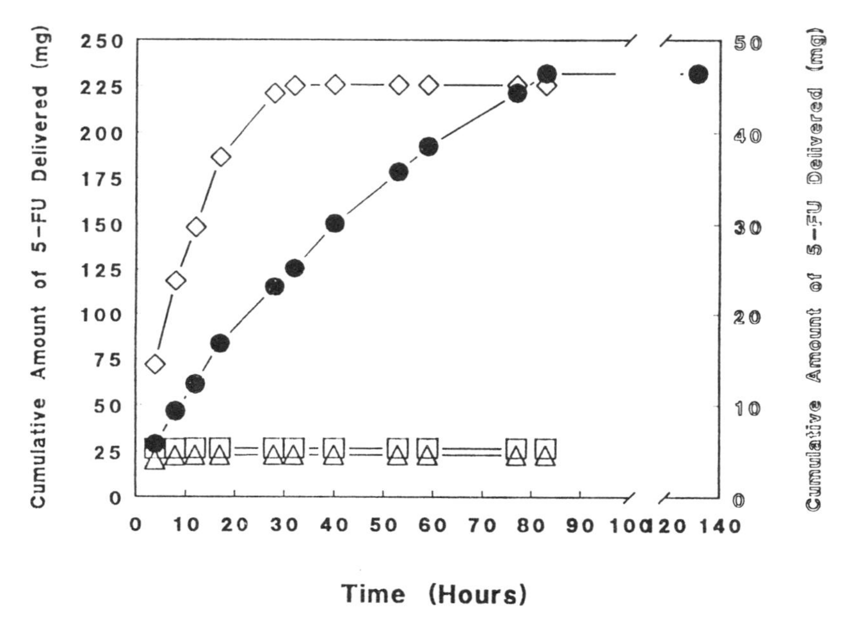


**FIGURE 15.2**
Cumulative amount of 5-FU delivered from fibrin sealant clots under limited-sink conditions. Fibrin sealant clots with a volume of 400 $\mu$L and containing various amounts of 5-FU were placed in 2 mL of buffer that was changed every twenty-four hours. The concentration of 5-FU released into the eluate was determined spectrophotometrically, and the total mass of 5-FU within the eluate calculated. (△): FS with 7 mg of aqueous 5-FU, (□): FS with 7 mg of anhydrous 5-FU, (◇): FS with 50 mg of anhydrous 5-FU, (¢ ): FS with 200 mg of anhydrous 5-FU. Values for the first three groups are plotted against the right side *Y*-axis, while values for the last group are plotted against the left side *Y*-axis.

tinued for eight and twelve hours for clots containing 50 and 200 mg of 5-FU respectively (Figure 15.3).

## DISCUSSION

The advantages of local or regional delivery of antiproliferative drugs include the ability to deliver high concentrations of the drugs for prolonged periods while maintaining low systemic concentrations. Using a "therapeutic implant" consisting of a protein gel, epinephrine, and an antiproliferative compound, local treatment of basal cell carcinoma [4,6], psoriasis [5], condylomata acuminata [15], and prostate cancer [10] has been performed with generally successful results. In C3H mice, these implants maintained an intralesional concentration of methotrexate that was thirty-two times greater than the systemic concentration [8]. These implants do not contain fibrinogen, which may have properties, including its adhesive and hemostatic activities, that would enhance the therapeutic efficacy of intralesional or supralesional therapy.

In order to determine if a fibrinogen-based delivery system might be practical, the duration of delivery of the antiproliferative compound 5-FU from fibrin sealant was investigated. It was determined that with small (400 μL) quantities of fibrin sealant, a total of 200 mg of 5-FU could be delivered. To attain these high loading levels, the anhydrous form of the drug was required due to the low solubility of 5-FU at physiological pH. The duration of delivery varied from twelve to eighty hours, depending upon the volume of the eluate and the presence or absence of agitation. While it is currently unknown whether the "limited-sink" or "infinite-sink" model will most closely model the situation in vivo, this range of delivery times would seem to be clinically

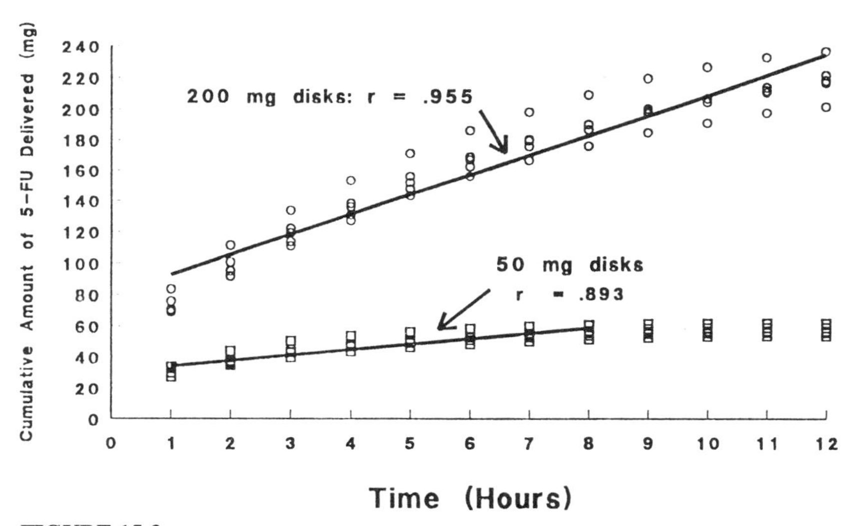


**FIGURE 15.3**
Cumulative amount of 5-FU delivered from fibrin sealant clots under infinite-sink conditions. Fibrin sealant clots with a volume of 400 μL and containing various amounts of 5-FU were placed in 50 mL of buffer that was continuously agitated and sampled every hour. The concentration of 5-FU released into the eluate was determined spectrophotometrically, and the total mass of 5-FU within the eluate calculated. (□): FS with 50 mg of anhydrous 5-FU, (○): FS with 200 mg of anhydrous 5-FU.

useful, as they lie within the range of the times reported for the previously mentioned treatment [8]. In addition, experience with fibrinogen-based delivery of antibiotics under limited- and infinite-sink delivery systems in vitro and in vivo, suggest that the limited-sink in vitro tests produce results closest to the in vivo results [16].

Results of tests of the sensitivity of several murine and human tumor cell lines to 5-FU indicate that the concentrations of 5-FU achieved in the limited-sink experiments exceeded the levels required to inhibit 95% of cell growth in vitro (data not shown). In a preliminary experiment, a single injection of FS + 5-FU into subcutaneous murine renal carcinoma tumors resulted in a rapid reduction in tumor volume, indicating that antiproliferative compounds can be delivered from FS in vivo (data not shown).

## CONCLUSIONS

Fibrinogen which has unique hemostatic and adhesive properties has been proposed as a delivery vehicle for drugs and biologics. These properties suggest that fibrin sealant might serve as a useful delivery vehicle for the delivery of antiproliferative compounds for the local/regional treatment of cancer or other neoplasms. It has been shown that one such drug, 5-FU, can be formulated into fibrin sealant in a manner that results in the delivery of the drug in a linear fashion between 6 to 80 hours. In a limited-sink experiment analogous to injection into a defined tumor mass, the levels of drug reached were greater than those required to inhibit the growth of several human and murine tumor cell lines, and a rapid tumor debulking was attained in vivo with a single injection of FS + 5-FU. The results indicate that fibrin sealant may be capable of serving as a delivery system for local/regional therapy of neoplasms in vivo.

## ACKNOWLEDGEMENTS

The authors wish to thank Dr. R. Wiltrout for his generous gift of the RENCA cell line and 5-FU.

## REFERENCES

1. Jain, R. Therapeutic implications of tumor physiology. *Current Opinions in Oncology,* 3:1105, 1991.
2. Eskey, C., Koretsky, A., Domach, M., Jain, R. 2H-nuclear magnetic resonance

imaging of tumor blood flow: Spatial and temporal heterogeneity in a tissue-isolated mammary adenocarcinoma. *Can. Res.*, 52:6010, 1992.

3. Goetz, A., Messmer, K., Kastenbauer, E., Jain, R. Interstitial hypertension in head and neck tumors in patients: Correlation with tumor size. *Can. Res.*, 52:7, 1992.
4. Promising new approaches to carcinoma treatment. *Skin and Allergy News*, 22:1, 1991.
5. Many innovative therapies for psoriasis hold promise. *Skin and Allergy News*, 22:1, 1991.
6. Orenberg, E., Miller, B., Greenway, H., Koperski, J., Lowe, N., Rosen, T., Brown, D., Inui, M., Korey, A., Luck, E. The effect of intralesional 5-Fluorouracil therapeutic implant (MPI 5003) for treatment of basal cell carcinoma. *J. Amer. Acad. of Derm.*, 27:723, 1992.
7. Miller, B., Greenway, H., Koperski, J., Lowe, N., Rosen, T., Luck, E., Brown, D., Orenberg, E. Basal cell carcinomas histologically resolved after treatment with intralesional 5-Fluorouracil therapeutic implant. *Proc. Amer. Assoc. Cancer Res.* 32:420 (Abstract #2496), 1991.
8. Yu, N., Palecek, J., Luck, E., Brown, D., Orenberg, E., Lalakea, L. Shinn, J. Pharmacokinetics and clinical application of the intralesional methotrexate therapeutic implant. *Proc. of ASCO*, 11:100 (Abstract #222), 1992.
9. Yu, N., Palecek, J., Luck, E., Brown, D. Comparison of antitumor effects of treatment sequence of Fluorouracil (FU) and Cisplatin (Pt) therapeutic implants in a mouse tumor model. *Proc. of ASCO*, 11:100 (Abstract #223), 1992.
10. Matrix Pharmaceuticels, Inc. *F-D-C Reports – "The Pink Sheet"* T&G-15 1993.
11. Saltz, R., Sierra, D., Feldman, D., Bartczak-Saltz, M., Dimick, A., Vasconez, L. O. Experimental and clinical applications of fibrin glue. *Plast. Reconstr. Surg.* 88:1005, 1991.
12. Sierra, D. Fibrin sealant adhesive systems: A review of their chemistry, material properties and clinical applications. *J. Biomater. Appl.*, 7:309, 1993.
13. Futami, H., Jansen, R., MacPhee, M. J., Keller, J., McCormick, K., Longo, D. L., Oppenheim, J. J., Ruscetti, F. W., Wiltrout, R. H. Chemoprotective effects of recombinant human IL-la in cyclophosphamide-treated normal and tumor-bearing mice. Protection from acute toxicity, hematological effects, development of late mortality, and enhanced therapeutic efficacy. *J. Immunol.*, 45:4121, 1990.
14. Fricke, W., Lamb, M. Viral safety of clotting factor concentrates. *Sem. Thromb. Hemostas.*, 19:56, 1993.
15. Conant, M., Beutner, K., Greene, I., Miller, B., Eron, L., Skinner, R., Buntin, D., Parish, L., Reihman, R., Thein, S., McCarty, J., Lang, W., Korey, A., Orenberg, E. Treatment of condylomata acuminate with intralesional 5-Fluorouracil therapeutic implant (MPI 5003). *Clin. Res.* 39:818A (Abstract), 1992.
16. MacPhee, M., Nunez, H. A., Hennings, R., Campagna, A., Harding, S., Drohan, W. Sustained release in vitro and in vivo of antibiotics from fibrin sealant. *Surgical Adhesives and Sealants: Current Technology and Applications.* D.H. Sierra and R. Saltz., eds. Technomic Publishing Co., Lancaster, PA 1996.

# *Chapter 16: Experimental and Clinical Considerations: Craniofacial Surgery and Bone Metabolism*

H. C. VASCONEZ and J. B. RODGERS

As craniofacial surgery has progressed, several initial problems have been solved while others remain, and still others are continually being discovered. There have been great demonstrations of wide mobilization of cranio-orbital bone segments to correct major deformity. However, in the process of such wide mobilization are other defects left that can also cause a deformity or dysfunction? The success of using rigid fixation in both congenital and traumatic craniomaxillofacial surgery has been noted. The diversity and versatility of the fixation implants have been greatly improved.

However, excessively rigid fixation in infants or growing patients may be restrictive or deleterious to normal growth and development. The use of bone grafts, increasingly of membranous origin, has become more and more popular for filling defects, providing stronger support, and promoting better contour. However, its predictability with respect to remodeling and resorption is still quite inadequate.

As a better understanding of normal and abnormal mechanisms of bone healing and regeneration is acquired, researchers are better equipped to answer some of the questions raised. New questions can now be posed for continued research. Research began with the study of the effects of fibrin glue in craniofacial surgery by trying to harness its hemostatic qualities during procedures tending towards large blood loss. Many authors in other fields have reported on the treatment of bleeding problems with preparations of fibrinogen-rich solutions. Rousou reported on the use of fibrin glue as an effective agent for nonsuturable, intraoperative bleeding in cardiac surgery [1]. Koveker used fibrin glue to coat and seal vascular grafts and noted less leakage [2]. Many anecdotal cases have been reported using fibrin glue to control intractable bleeding in splenic and hepatic injuries, resection of cranial tumors, renal and prostatic surgery, and others. Grimm has described the utility of fibrin glue in hemophiliacs who undergo dental or oral surgery [3].

We compared fibrin glue to the commonly-used hemostatic agent in craniofacial and bone surgery: bone wax. The tendency for bone wax to remain for prolonged periods of time was observed, and infections that were probably caused or aided by bone wax were noted. Fibrin glue compared to bone wax in split-thickness defects of the rat calvarium was investigated. Homologous rat plasma was used to prepare fibrin glue.

Female Wistar rats weighing 250 grams were divided into five groups of seven each (incision only, defect only, defect + fibrin glue, defect + bone wax, and defect + fibrin glue + bone chips). The rats were sacrificed at 1, 3, and 5 weeks, and tetracycline labeling was used to follow bone mineralization and growth by histomorphometry.

It was difficult to quantify hemorrhage or hemostasis but histologically, the bone wax and fibrin glue groups had much less hematoma formation than the control group. The fibrin glue group showed greater vascularity and more abundant bone growth than the bone wax group. The bone wax specimens displayed granuloma formation, hypocellularity, and actual necrosis of bone.

Bosch [4] showed that homologous, as opposed to heterologous, fibrin glue stimulated bone healing [4]. He further demonstrated that greater vascularity and new bone growth occur with fibrin glue in the presence of denatured, heterologous Kiel® bone graft, which has little or no osteogenic potential. Meyers showed the effects of fibrin glue in the repair of osteochondral fracture fragments [5]. The healing of osteochondral fracture fragments in a dog model compared fixation with glue or with pins. He reported the osseous repair to be faster and more complete with fibrin glue.

Albrektsson et al. took a dissenting opinion on fibrin glue. They showed a tendency toward less bone growth when compared to controls that contained added autologous blood and bone marrow cells [6]. The controls soon produced a fibrin matrix containing osteogenic cells and probably incorporating mitogenic factors that can stimulate osteogenesis. Their control group was more in line with an experimental group. Nevertheless, it brought up the subjects of osteogenic potential and bone growth factors in certain parts of the bone matrix, primarily the demineralized portion.

In using a rabbit cranium model for split-thickness defect repair, a technical problem developed in the rabbit with the production of autologous fibrin glue. The low yield of fibrinogen was because of the rabbit species, a fact noted by other researchers. The Weis-Fogh technique was modified and adequate amounts of fibrin adhesive were obtained from small amounts of rabbit plasma [7]. We performed 15 $mm^2$ split-cranial defects in the rabbit and divided them into four groups of twelve rabbits each (no treatment, fibrin glue, plasma supernatant or bone wax). Again there was rapid and satisfactory hemostasis achieved in both the fibrin-glue and bone-wax groups. Although the histomorphometric analysis is not complete, the fibrin-glue groups displayed greater early vascular and cellular response than the other three groups.

Animals in all groups were completely healed after eight weeks. In fact, during the first two weeks the amount of osteoid (O.Ar/B.Ar) and density of osteoblasts (# of Ob./$\mu$m bone surface) decreased significantly ($p = .001$) (Figure 16.1). During the same period, the osteoclast density (# of Oc./$\mu$m bone surface) increased significantly ($p = .002$) (see Figure 16.2). Defects treated with fibrin glue had significantly ($p = .03$) higher osteoclast density at two weeks.

This suggests that the angiogenesis ascribed to the presence of fibrin glue influences the attraction of osteoclasts to the local site, resulting in more rapid remodeling of new woven bone to lamellar bone (see Figure 16.3 and Table 16.1). It should be emphasized that these were split-thickness cranial defects and not full-thickness critical size defects that would not heal if left untreated.

Almost thirty years ago, Urist proposed the concept of bone formation by autoinduction [8]. The concepts of osteoinduction and osteoconduction are now used very commonly and are beginning to be understood. He also

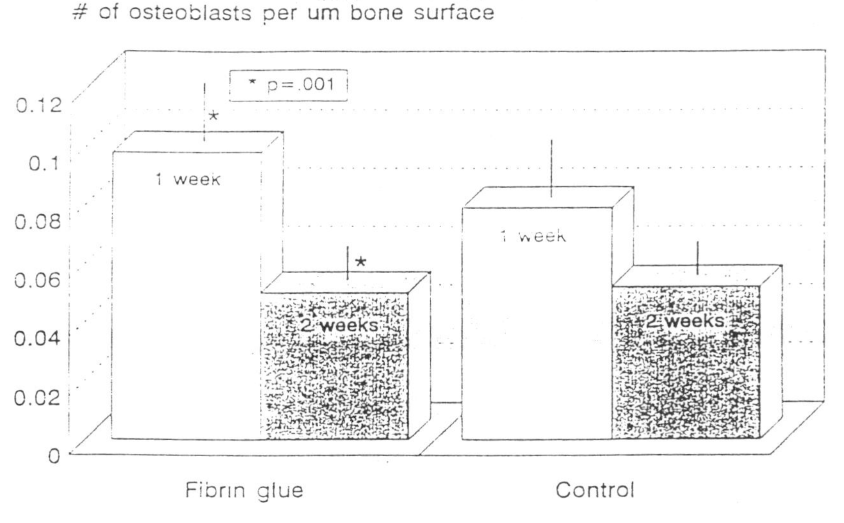


**FIGURE 16.1**
Osteoblast numbers.

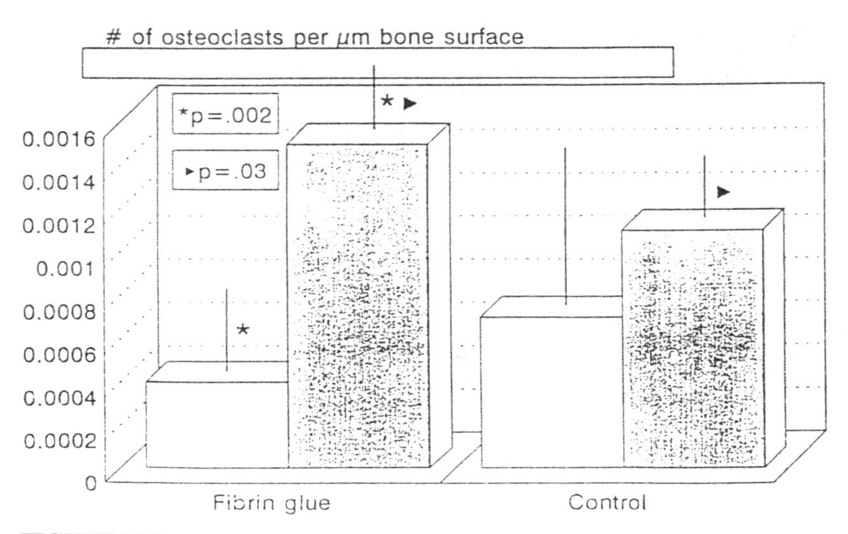


**FIGURE 16.2**
Osteoclast numbers.

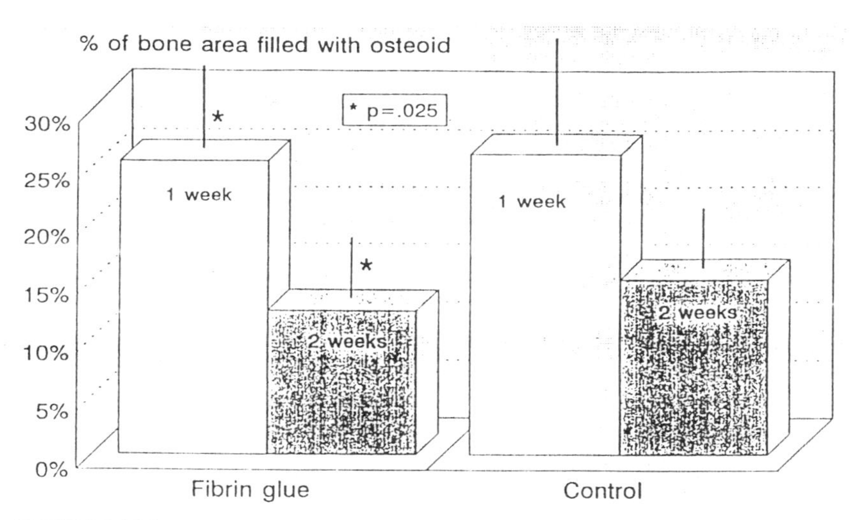


**FIGURE 16.3**
Osteoid production.

***Table 16.1.*** *Parameters of bone healing.*

| Time | Group | *n* | O.Ar./ B.Ar. (% ±S.D.) | N. Ob./μm (±S.D.) | N. Oc./μm (±S.D.) | Osteoid thickness (μm) (±S.D.) |
|---|---|---|---|---|---|---|
| 1 wk | Fibrin glue | 3 | 25.4 ± 8.52 | 0.098 ± 0.020 | 0.0004 ± 0.0004 | 9.15 ± 1.6 |
| 2 wks | Fibrin glue | 6 | 12.4 ± 5.49 | 0.050 ± 0.009 | 0.0015 ± 0.0003 | 7.51 ± 1.7 |
| 1 wk | Control | 3 | 26.0 ± 15.01 | 0.079 ± 0.022 | 0.0007 ± 0.0007 | 10.99 ± 1.8 |
| 2 wks | Control | 8 | 15.1 ± 8.12 | 0.0052 ± 0.0015 | 0.0011 ± 0.0003 | 12.21 ± 10.7 |

introduced a product derived from demineralized bovine bone matrix that he termed "bone morphogenetic protein." These very potent cytokines have been further purified and cDNA clones have been obtained to encode individual proteins. They can subsequently be expressed in recombinant systems to produce highly purified human proteins.

There are at least seven BMPs known and all are members of the TGF-β superfamily. Work is being done with these and other growth factors to stimulate, modulate, and better understand bone healing and regeneration. In our laboratory, work continues to combine the positive effects of fibrin glue on angiogenesis and bone healing with the inclusion of these bone growth factors.

Much of this work is being done at a Veterans Administration hospital. The patients suffered wounds in military action or are civilians with healing and structural disorders resulting from trauma, cancer, or other debilitating diseases. Simple and effective means of promoting wound and bone healing are greatly needed in this patient population. Enhancement of revascularization and stimulated new bone growth in cases of large defects, nonunions or complicated fractures can provide a major decrease in morbidity and save money.

## REFERENCES

1. Rousou, J. A., Engelman, R. M., Breyer, R. H. Fibrin glue: An effective hemostatic agent for nonsuturable intraoperative bleeding. *Ann. Thorac. Surg.*, 38:409–410, 1984.
2. Koveker, G. Clinical application of fibrin glue in cardiovascular surgery. *Thorac. Cardiovasc. Surg.*, 30:228, 1982.
3. Grimm, G., Niekisch, R. Zur problematik eines hamophilie-dispensaires unter den bedingungen der fibrinklebung. *Z. Stomatol.*, 83:239, 1986.

4. Bosch, P., Lintner, F., Arbes, H., Brand, G. Experimental investigations of the effect of the fibrin adhesive on the Kiel® heterologous bone graft. *Arch. Orthop. Trauma Surg.* 96:177–185, 1980.
5. Meyers, M. H., Herron, M. A fibrin adhesive seal for the repair of osteochondral fracture fragments. *Clin. Orthop.*, 182:258–263, 1984.
6. Albrektsson, T., Bach, A., Edshage, S., Jönsson, A. Fibrin adhesive system (FAS) influence on bone healing rate. *Acta. Orthop. Scand.*, 53:757–763, 1982.
7. Weis-Fogh, U. S. Fibrinogen prepared from small blood samples for autologous use in a tissue adhesive system. *Eur. Surg. Res.*, 20:381–389, 1988.
8. Urist, M. R. Bone: Formation by autoinduction. *Science*, 150:893–899, 1965.

# SECTION IV

# CLINICAL APPLICATIONS AND INVESTIGATIONS

# *Chapter 17: Fibrin Sealant and the U.S. Food and Drug Administration Review Process*

W. A. FRICKE

## INTRODUCTION

The United States Food and Drug Administration (FDA) is responsible for assuring the safety and efficacy of all drugs and biologics sold in the United States. The regulatory authority for drugs is contained in the Federal Food, Drug, and Cosmetic (FD&C) Act, and for biologics in the Public Health Service (PHS) Act. The FD&C Act defines drugs as "articles intended for use in the diagnosis, cure, mitigation, treatment, or prevention of disease in man or other animals . . . and intended to affect the structure or any function of the body of man . . ." [1]. The PHS Act defines a biologic as ". . . any virus, therapeutic serum, toxin, antitoxin, vaccine, blood, blood component or derivative, allergenic product, or analogous product . . . applicable to the prevention, treatment, or cure of diseases or injuries of man . . ." [2]. Although there are similarities between the definitions of drugs and of biologics, there are important differences between them.

The most fundamental of these is that a drug is typically a chemical entity that can be well-characterized with respect to its physical attributes, including its structure. A biologic, on the other hand, is typically a complex mixture of components that cannot be successfully separated and characterized. The inability to fully characterize the final product has required the regulation of biologics to rely more heavily on in-process testing and validation of production to assure product safety, potency, and consistency rather than on final product testing.

The process of licensure of biologics is similar to that for drug approval. In both cases an investigational new drug application (IND) must be filed, clinical trials performed, and an application for licensure or approval submitted to the FDA. In the case of biologics, the application for licensure is a product license application (PLA), whereas drugs require the submission of a new drug application (NDA). In addition, biologics require that the manufacturing establishment also be licensed through the submission of an establishment license application (ELA) (preparation and review of ELAs will not be discussed here). For both drugs and biologics, the safety, purity, potency, and efficacy of the product must be established. The following review will focus on the licensing process for biologics with emphasis on the design and execution of clinical trials. Issues that are relevant to clinical trials of fibrin sealant will be discussed.

## INVESTIGATIONAL NEW DRUGS

All unlicensed and licensed drugs being tested for a new indication are considered investigational and cannot be marketed in interstate commerce. A sponsor wishing to perform a clinical trial on a new drug that will involve shipping the drug across state lines must submit a "Notice of Claimed Investigational Exemption for a New Drug," commonly known as an IND. The sponsor may begin the study thirty days from the date of the submission, providing the FDA does not place the IND on "hold." This is usually done only when there are significant questions regarding the safety of the drug or the soundness of the proposed clinical trial.

Primary concerns during the review of the IND are that adequate data have been provided to establish that a new drug is safe to use in clinical trials, and that the clinical trial to be performed will generate useful and acceptable data [3]. To accomplish these goals, the IND should include a description of the preparation of the drug and of all preclinical testing or other use of the drug (Table 17.1). The IND should describe the chemistry,

***Table 17.1.*** *IND content and format.*

| |
|---|
| **Cover Sheet:** Identify sponsor, IRB Statement, general administration |
| **Introductory Statement:** Name of drug, mechanism of action, marketing history, brief description of clinical trial. |
| **Investigator's Brochure:** Summary of safety and clinical data. |
| **Protocols:** Plan for clinical investigation. |
| **Chemistry, Manufacturing, and Controls:** Describes the composition, method of manufacture, and quality control measures. |
| **Pharmacology and Toxicology:** Describes the studies and results upon which the sponsor has determined it is reasonably safe to conduct the clinical trials. |
| **Previous Human Experience:** Summary of other use. |
| **Additional Information:** Dependence/abuse potential, radioactive drug information. |

manufacturing, and control procedures involved in making the drug. The drug should be characterized with respect to its physical properties, and the final container material should be described, including all excipients. Finally, the proposed clinical use and an outline of the clinical trials intended to demonstrate the drug's efficacy and safety should be included.

The description of the preparation of the drug is particularly important in biologics because of the general inability to precisely characterize these types of products. For a plasma-derived product, the collection, storage, and fractionation of the plasma should be described. This includes the specific conditions under which this is done, the chemicals used in processing, and occasionally, some of the equipment used. The reviewer of a well-written IND should be able to determine aspects of manufacturing, such as temperature, pH, processing time, chemicals added, and filters and chromatography columns used. The product testing and specifications for in-process material at each step of manufacturing and on the final product should also be described.

An IND for a recombinant protein must include a description of the cloning of the gene, construction of the plasmid, the cell in which the protein is produced, the culture conditions, the purification process, and product testing. A successful IND will provide adequate biochemical and molecular biologic evidence of safety.

Toxicologic studies are usually performed on new products before the IND is submitted. These studies typically involve several different animal species that receive large doses of the product. Adverse effects may be looked for through laboratory tests, clinical observations, or pathologic examination. These studies can be valuable in detecting toxicity of a new drug and in estimating the appropriate human dose. However, species differences may complicate the interpretation of the data generated. One species may react to a drug that other species, including humans, may not react to. None of the species tested may react to a drug that has significant toxicity for humans. Interpretation of toxicity test results can also be complicated by the fact that the doses used are usually much higher than those that would ever be used in humans; thus the relevance of adverse reactions in the animals to toxicity in humans is often unclear.

A description of the proposed clinical trials should also be submitted. Typically, clinical trials are divided into three phases [4]. Phase 1 is primarily intended to assess the safety and pharmacokinetics of the drug. These trials may be done on normal volunteers or on the patient population to be studied. Data from the phase 1 trial may be used to design a phase 2 study intended primarily to demonstrate the efficacy of the drug on a designated patient population. Efficacy and safety are the primary objectives of a phase 2 study. In some situations a phase 2 trial may be the "pivotal" trial used to support licensure.

Phase 3 trials are typically larger than phase 2 and are intended to generate additional efficacy and safety data. These data are used to supplement the data gathered in phase 2 and provide an adequate basis for labeling. In some instances, a phase 4 trial may be performed. Phase 4 trials are done after the licensure of a drug and are intended to provide additional data or to answer any remaining questions regarding use of the drug. This may be related to adverse reactions or use in a particular patient group.

Many INDs include a fairly detailed plan for a phase 1 trial but, as would be expected, include only a general outline for phases 2 and 3. Following completion of phase 1, a more specific plan for phase 2 is submitted. Often this is done following a meeting with the FDA in which the details of the proposed trial are discussed. These may include not only the design, but also the conduct of the trial, the specific statistical analyses that will be used, and criterion (criteria) of efficacy. Important issues that must be settled include blinding, the nature of the placebo, if used, interim analyses, monitoring, and criteria for early stopping.

Several important points should be made about efficacy trials. First, the end points should be specified and well-defined. End points such as "improved quality of life" or "general feeling of well-being" are vague, subjective, and difficult to quantitate. On the other hand, end points such as the number of infections, the occurrence of deep-vein thrombosis, or disease-free survival, lend themselves better to standardization and objective assessment. Obviously, the sponsor, clinical investigator, and the FDA should be in agreement about the exact objectives of the trial.

Second, methods of evaluating each patient should be agreed upon. Usually, a combination of laboratory and clinical findings is used to support this assessment. For instance, venography would be a possible measurement for assessing the status of patients in a trial of a drug intended to prevent deep-vein thrombosis. In contrast, clinical observation, although it might provide some useful information, would not be acceptable for such an evaluation. Third, the number of end points should be limited. Usually one, or at most two, primary end points are used.

One of the difficulties with multiple end points is that this increases the number of subgroups and can significantly compromise the validity of the outcome. In addition, one to three secondary end points that are in some way related to the primary end points or the mechanism of action of the drug may be included. For example, mortality from cardiovascular disease could be the primary end point for a drug used to treat myocardial infarction. Secondary end points could then be overall mortality or clot lysis, as in the case of a thrombolytic agent. And, fourth, the end points must have clinical significance in that the drug must be shown to confer some clinical benefit on the patient. This is a more difficult area because our perceptions of what constitutes clinical benefit may vary. Improvement in hemoglobin concentration in patients treated with erythropoietin could be seen as having clinical significance for the patient, but perhaps only if the patient would require blood transfusion without that improvement.

The FDA recognizes the difficulty manufacturers face in preparing INDs and has issued a variety of "Guidelines" and "Points to Consider" that can be used to develop and test their products. These documents offer guidance and suggestions on issues regarded as important by the FDA. The FDA also recognizes that the production process of a drug may be modified during its development and testing in order to optimize yield, improve safety, or enhance some other characteristic. The manufacturing process for a drug tested in phase 1 may differ somewhat from the process used in phases 2 or 3, although changes that are likely to affect safety or efficacy will probably require repetition of earlier clinical trials to validate changes.

## PRODUCT LICENSE APPLICATION

A product license application is submitted to the Center for Biologic Evaluation and Research (CBER) following the completion of the clinical trials. The PLA should contain complete and detailed information about product manufacturing, testing, safety, and efficacy. The manufacturing process should describe the steps used to create the product for which the license is being applied; and the pivotal clinical trials should have been performed using the drug product manufactured by that process.

The information about product manufacturing included in a PLA is similar to that in an IND, although a PLA is typically more comprehensive [5]. In addition to a description of each step in processing, each step is also validated. That is, data are supplied to show that each step does what it purports to do every time it is performed. The result is that the data support the lot-to-lot consistency of the product. The PLA also includes considerable product characterization data. For a plasma-derived product this usually includes biochemical and immunologic data.

Recombinant products, in addition, have data on the cells used in production and the molecular biology of the product. The type of data submitted may include immunoblots, chromatograms, peptide maps, amino acid composition, isoelectric focussing patterns, glycosylation, circular dichroism/optical rotatory dispersion, potency, and immunogenicity data. Cells and culture media used in the production of recombinant proteins must also be tested for the presence of endogenous viruses and for bacteria, fungi, and mycoplasma. Moreover, at various stages the cells may be tested to establish their freedom from adventitious agents, their identity, their integrity, and the integrity of the construct used in transection [6,7].

An additional important part of the PLA submission is data supporting the stability of the product over time. Obviously, for a product to be economically viable it must have a reasonable shelf life or dating period. This issue is addressed in studies in which the product is stored at relevant temperatures and tested periodically for stability. Parameters may include, in addition to activity, other measures of degradation such as aggregation or fragmentation. Many plasma-derived products are licensed to be stored at 2–8°C for several years, although some may also be stored at room temperature for shorter periods of time. For lyophilized products, stability data is also usually generated on the reconstituted product.

Results of the clinical trials should also be included in the PLA. The submission should give complete details of the pharmacokinetics and pharmacodynamics of the drug. Important drug interactions, if known, should be included. Results of the phase 2 and phase 3 trials should also be presented. As with the other sections of a PLA, complete details of the trials should be provided. The total number of patients enrolled should be stated, the number of patients treated, and the number of those who dropped out, were excluded, or were otherwise not included in the final efficacy evaluation. The results should be analyzed by appropriate statistical methods.

One potentially contentious issue that occasionally arises in analyzing clinical trials is subgroup analysis. As a general rule if a subgroup of patients was not defined prospectively as one in which efficacy would be tested, then any benefit seen in the subgroup is not sufficient to demonstrate efficacy. In other words, it is not valid to claim efficacy for a subgroup of patients identified retrospectively as having received benefit from the drug. If it appears that a group of patients within the trial, but not identified prospectively, has benefitted from the therapy, then this hypothesis should be tested prospectively in a new trial.

One of the concerns about subgroup analysis is bias. Bias is a type of systematic error that occurs in a study either intentionally or unintentionally. It is the major reason why studies should be blinded. There are many sources of bias. These include extrapolation of data from one patient population to another, or larger, patient group; patient selection bias; observer bias; and trials that are observational, case-controlled, retrospective, or uncontrolled. Bias that is likely to be introduced into subgroup analysis comes from the retrospective selection of patients for the subgroup. Despite efforts to avoid it, retrospective selection of patients may favor inclusion of patients who benefitted from the therapy and thus distort the outcome of the trial.

## FIBRIN SEALANT

This brief review of the licensing process for biologics was intended to set the background for a discussion of fibrin sealant. Fibrin sealant is typical of biologics in that it is a complex mixture of proteins, many of which cannot be easily characterized. The availability of sophisticated purification procedures makes it possible to remove all the extraneous proteins from the preparation, but this is not practical and would reduce the production yield and drive up costs.

The same principles apply to the licensure of fibrin sealant as to all other biologics; namely, safety and efficacy must be established through control of the manufacturing process by product testing and through clinical trials. As with all plasma-derived products, an important safety concern with fibrin sealant is transmission of blood-borne viruses, such as hepatitis B (HBV), hepatitis C (HCV), and human immunodeficiency virus (HIV). Current donor screening and testing have reduced to very low levels the risk for transmission of these viruses by blood transfusion [8]. However, the large number of donors who contribute to a pool of plasma used in making plasma derivatives greatly increases the likelihood that the pool will contain infectious viruses. For this reason, all plasma-derived products include in their manufacturing process steps that will remove or inactivate contaminating viruses.

Inactivation methods currently in use include heating the lyophilized final product, heating the product in solution or in the presence of increased moisture, and treating the product with mixtures of solvents and detergents. Various types of affinity chromatography may also be used to remove viruses, while at the same time purifying the protein of interest.

Evaluating the efficacy of the viral removal/inactivation methods is problematic. Clinical safety studies have been done in which hemophiliacs who have never received blood products are exposed to the treated product and then tested regularly for signs of infection. These trials are difficult to do because they require several years for completion and because these so-called ''naive'' patients are uncommon. Alternatively, the removal/inactivation procedure can be tested in vitro.

Unfortunately, of the viruses listed above that are infectious to man, only HIV can be grown in culture. Thus, surrogate or marker viruses are used for HBV and HCV. In a typical experiment, a known amount of the marker virus is added to in-process material prior to the step of interest and the amount of virus present before and after the step is determined. The difference in amount of the initial and remaining virus is a measure of the ability of the process to eliminate infectious virus from the product. A major difficulty with this approach is the inability to correlate elimination of a surrogate virus from the product with a finite reduction in risk of transmission of infectious virus to recipients of the product. Nonetheless, this approach has value in that it can be used to validate the elimination method.

Another major issue is the efficacy of fibrin sealant. Within this issue are two questions: (1) Is the product efficacious, and, if so, for what indications? (2) What are the contributions to efficacy of the various components of the product? As has already been discussed, efficacy should be demonstrated through a randomized, controlled, blinded clinical trial. Inability to blind the operator is a potential problem in some situations, although this can be partially compensated for by having a second, blinded person do the efficacy evaluation.

The appropriate end points obviously depend upon the purpose of the trial. In wound healing or tissue adhesions, the strength, cosmetic result, or integrity of the wound or joint may be reasonable end points. In hemostasis, possible end points include blood loss, transfusion requirements or time to hemostasis.

The end points chosen should clearly signify clinical benefit to the patient. For instance, it is questionable if there is a statistically significant decrease in blood loss from 30 mL to 10 mL during a procedure without necessarily improving the outcome. Fibrin sealant might eliminate the need for staples or suture in some situations. However, it would be necessary to perform a clinical trial that would demonstrate that this is the case and that the outcome is at least equivalent to the current practice.

The method of application of fibrin sealant is also a potential problem. It may be applied directly using a syringelike spray device or by using a carrier, such as collagen or cellulose sponges. A clinical trial should be designed to demonstrate the importance or necessity, if any, of the method of application. This requires that the contribution of the carrier to the clinical effect be established. As an example, if the purpose of the trial is to demonstrate hemostasis, then a three-arm trial comparing fibrin sealant plus the carrier to fibrin sealant alone and to the carrier alone should be done.

The wide variety of procedures and circumstances in which fibrin sealant could be used raises the issue of how broadly to write the indications and uses sections of the package circular. Ideally, adequate and well-controlled clinical trials should be performed for every licensed indication. Indications for hemostasis in cardiovascular surgery, orthopedic surgery, or burn excision require trials in each of those settings. Similarly, indications for use as a tissue adhesive in neurosurgery, otologic surgery, or plastic surgery require trials in each of those situations.

The reason for requiring a trial in each area is that the efficacy and safety may differ depending upon the specific use and setting. Rapid hemostasis with a decreased need for transfusions and few adverse reactions may be found in burn excision, whereas the hemostatic benefit may be much less or the incidence of adverse reactions much higher in orthopedic surgery. On the other hand, practical considerations make it unlikely that good clinical trials will ever be performed in all of the situations in which fibrin sealant might be of value. A reasonable compromise may be to require one or more well-done, controlled, clinical trial for each broad indication, such as hemostasis or wound healing, and encourage the accumulation of safety and efficacy data for all other possible uses.

Fibrin sealant is a combination product. The active ingredients include fibrinogen-thrombin preparations, Factor XIII, plasminogen, fibronectin, calcium, and in some formulations, aprotinin. This raises the second major question. What are the contributions of the various active ingredients? The regulations require that each claimed active ingredient of a combination product must be shown to make a contribution to the effect of the final product [9,10]. If a protein copurifies with a component for which a claimed contribution is made, then the copurifying protein does not necessarily have to be removed.

No claim can be made for the protein's contribution to the efficacy of the product, and no specifications can be sent for the amounts of the protein in the product. For instance, fibronectin and Factor XIII tend to copurify with fibrinogen. As long as the manufacturer does not claim that either protein contributes to efficacy then there is no need to specify that certain amounts of these proteins must be in the product.

However, if the manufacturer claims that these proteins, whether they copurify or not, are important to the effect of the product or that they must be present in certain amounts, then their contribution to efficacy must be demonstrated. This may be done with appropriate experimental design in clinical studies by using the product with and without each active ingredient. Under suitable circumstances, appropriate animal studies of such design may be acceptable for demonstrating the contribution.

There is, however, flexibility in the FDA's application of this regulation to fibrin sealant. Since the activity of the product lies in its ability to form a fibrin clot, then clearly both the fibrinogen and the thrombin must be present, and it would not be necessary to show that a clot only forms if both are present. However, the roles of the other ingredients are less clear.

Both calcium and Factor XIII are necessary if the fibrin monomers in the clot are to be crosslinked, but the necessity for cross-linking is uncertain. This could be shown in a study that demonstrates an increased incidence of rebleeding when product showing the importance of the other components should be done. In an ideal world, these studies would be done in patients. However, the FDA also recognizes that testing all the combinations of product with and without the various components would be a difficult task. Therefore, under appropriate circumstances, well-controlled animal experiments that clearly demonstrate a clinically relevant contribution of these ingredients could substitute for studies in humans.

## CONCLUSION

The goal of the drug-review process is to determine safety and efficacy for which there are no simple or easy tests. Safety must be established through strict control of the manufacturing process and through testing in vitro, in animals, and in clinical trials. Before a new drug reaches the IND stage, much of the safety testing must have already been completed, and there must be enough data to insure that giving the drug to humans does not pose an unreasonable risk. An IND must also contain a proposed clinical study that is likely to generate data that will be adequate to support licensure of the product.

The PLA can be submitted after the manufacturing process is established and the clinical trials are completed. It should contain detailed information about the drug's manufacturing process and the drug's safety and efficacy.

An adequately performed and fully analyzed clinical trial is often fundamental to the success of the application. The key elements in designing and conducting a clinical trial include a clearly stated purpose, one or two well-defined end points that have clinical significance, acceptable methods of evaluating the outcome, and a design that minimizes bias. Bias can be limited through prospective studies that include randomization, blinding, and use of placebo controls. Early and frequent contact between manufacturers and the FDA will often prevent problems and avoid delays in review and approval.

## REFERENCES


1. Food, Drug, and Cosmetic Act, Sec. 201(g)(1).
2. Public Health Service Act, Sec. 351(a).
3. 21 CFR 312.23.
4. 21 CFR 312.31.
5. 21 CFR 601.2.
6. Information Package for the Nucleic Acid Characterization of Host Cells Used in the Production of Recombinant DNA Products, Center for Biologics Evaluation and Research, 1992.
7. Points to Consider in the Characterization of Cell Lines used to Produce Biologicals, Center for Biologics Evaluation and Research, 1992.
8. Dodd, R. Y. The risk of transfusion-transmitted infection. *N. Engl. J. Med.*, 327:419–421, 1992.
9. 21 CFR 300.50(a).
10. 21 CFR 601.25(d)(4).

# *Chapter 18: Utilization of Fibrin Glue in Craniofacial and Facial Plastic Surgery*

D. MARCHAC

When fibrin glue (FG) first became available (Tissucol, Immuno AG, Vienna), its utilization was of great interest for plastic surgery.

In 1983, experience in the use of fibrin glue was presented to the French Society of Plastic and Reconstructive Surgery. At that time, FG was used mainly for application of full-thickness skin grafts of the face. It was learned rapidly that one has to apply a very thin layer to avoid creating a barrier. The percentage of full-take skin grafts seemed to improve. Fibrin glue was also tried for facelifts. The adherence was good and satisfactory results with a small number of patients were obtained. The use of fibrin glue for facelifts was abandoned, however, because of the need for large quantities to cover all the undermined areas. It was in 1986, when the spray system became available, that use was resumed for large, undermined areas and in particular for facelifts.

## THE USE OF SPRAYED FIBRIN GLUE IN FACELIFTS

The application is simple: after completion of undermining, fat removal, SMAS reshaping, and hemostasis is established, the skin flaps are put under tension. The key stitches are placed, but not tied; these are suspended on a hemostat. To facilitate precise adjustment, the two main key stitches are tied behind the ear and under the temporal hair. They are removed and left uncut after the skin adjustment has carefully been made. The skin flaps are then elevated with wide retractors and the undermined area is sprayed. One cc of fibrin glue for each side is used, under slow coagulation (thirty seconds) conditions.

As soon as the spraying is done, the surgeon carefully drapes the skin flap in the desired position. Care is taken to avoid folds, especially in the malar and temporal areas. The assistant then ties the knots and a final adjustment with sutures is performed; care is taken not to lift the glued flaps while suturing. If a separate short submental incision had been performed, a few drops of FG, rather than spray, are applied to the central neck portion before suturing.

No drains or dressings are used. The face is cleansed without rubbing; the hair washed, combed, and dried. The patients, with instructions to remain quiet and keep their chins up, are placed on clean towels.

There are two advantages to avoiding drainage and dressings: (1) reduction of post-surgical time by not putting on and removing the usual bulky, carefully arranged dressings; and (2) detection of swelling and hematomas is easier. When a hematoma occurs, the gluing of the flaps limits the area of expansion of the hematoma. It quickly produces an easy-to-detect bulge instead of the usual slow spreading of hematoma under the entire undermined area. A limited evacuation followed by compression usually solves the problem and reopenings are rare [1].

The early follow-up was very satisfactory; a greater number of patients, where fibrin glue was used, had limited edema and bruising in comparison to patients without FG. This allowed for faster recovery. Connell has said that this improvement was mostly due, in his opinion, to the absence of dressings [2]. He did not use dressings or glue on the incision.

A study of the effects of utilizing drains and dressings with and without FG was made. On ten patients, FG was applied on one side. No drains or dressings were used on either side. In five patients, the results were equivocal, with limited edema and bruising. In the five other patients, the results were always better on the side that was glued. One smoker had a significant retro-auricular slough on the nonglued side and a much smaller one on the glued side. Another patient had a small hematoma on the nonglued side, and none on the glued side. Two had more bruises and edema on the nonglued side. Although it was a short series, the use of fibrin glue was encouraging. Since 1986, it is used for all facelifts in our clinic.

A statistical analysis was performed on facelifts done before 1986. One hundred facelifts were performed without fibrin glue and 100 were performed with the use of sprayed fibrin glue [3]. This study reported that the incidence of large hematomas had significantly diminished and that the percentage of quick recovery with limited edema and bruising was higher.

There are two drawbacks to the use of fibrin glue. One is the slight loss of time due to the placement of long stay sutures, and the other is the cost of the fibrin glue, which is not negligible.

The use of sprayed fibrin glue in over 700 facelifts has shown no adverse reactions. One exception was a case of cervical edema and seroma collection in an area that corresponded to the area where the glue was sprayed. These problems disappeared without sequelae after a few weeks.

One of the main concerns is, of course, the risk of dissemination of transmitted diseases. No problem of this kind has been observed in this series. Distributors of fibrin glue have stated that all precautions are taken and in particular, that measures are taken to eliminate potential viruses.

An interesting recent development is the use of fibrin glue in frontal endoscopic surgery. Fibrin glue was previously used after coronal browlifts to obliterate the dead space, but the tension and positioning was determined by the strip of resected scalp. During an endoscopic frontal approach, fixation is difficult. A wide undermining is performed. Through minor incisions, the forehead, brows, and scalp are immobilized in the desired position.

Sprayed fibrin glue represents an excellent solution to this problem. Through the small scalp incisions, a thin, curved, bendable tube is inserted in the undermined space and fibrin glue is delivered through it. The forehead and temporal areas are immobilized for thirty seconds in the desired position. To insure better adhesion, undermining above the nerinstinum is preferred. No dressings are utilized. A longer follow-up (six months) is needed, but the repositioning seems stable.

## USE OF FIBRIN GLUE IN CRANIOFACIAL SURGERY

There are three major uses for fibrin glue in craniofacial surgery: (1) to glue patches or small bone fragments on the dura; (2) to mix with bone dust in order to occlude bony defects or irregularities; (3) to occlude dead spaces when replacing the skin [3].

Fluidtightness of the dura is essential. When defects of the dura must be repaired, a patch of periostium is used. Careful suturing is necessary, but gluing increases the tightness and facilitates the positioning.

Fibrin glue also facilitates the positioning of small bony fragments on areas where cranial defects and irregularities are present, as these fragments are too small to justify an osteosynthesis.

The mixture of fibrin glue and bone dust is one of the most interesting applications in craniofacial surgery. The bone dust is carefully collected while a surgeon is making the burr holes in the cranium. This dust is mixed with the same volume of fibrin glue. There are two ways to apply it. The first is to mix it with the fibrin glue and apply it to the full bony defects. This occludes the remnants of a frontal sinus or reconstructs the cranial base after correction of midline clefts. Thrombin is then applied and the mixture solidifies. The same method can be used for correction of small surface irregularities and filling of burr holes.

A second method of application is to mix the bone dust, fibrin glue, and thrombin and immediately spread them to a thickness of 2 or 3 mm. Solidification occurs quickly and it can then be cut with scissors to the desired shape and adjusted on the defect(s).

Despite these measures, nothing is as good as autogenous bone. The ideal is to split the calvaria. However, when that is not feasible, especially in children, the use of mixed bone dust and fibrin glue facilitates reossification. When full-thickness cranial grafts in children are taken, this technique is used. This offers the opportunity to verify in situ take.

## REFERENCES

1. Marchac, D., Pugash, E., Gault, D. The use of sprayed fibrin glue in facelifts. *Eur. J. Plast. Surg.* 10:139–143, 1987.
2. Connell, Bruce. Personal communication. 1993.
3. Marchac, D., Sandor, G. Facelifts and sprayed fibrin glue: An outcome analysis in 200 patients. *Brit. J. Plast. Surg.* ( in press, 1995).
4. Marchac, D., Renier, D. Fibrin glue in craniofacial surgery. *J. Craniofacial Surg.*, 11:32–44, 1990.

# *Chapter 19: Tissue Adhesives in Plastic and Reconstructive Surgery*

H. N. HIMEL

## INTRODUCTION

Two types of tissue adhesives have been widely used in plastic and reconstructive surgery: the acrylate adhesives and fibrin sealant [1–3]. Most reports describe the external application of the acrylate adhesives, while reports for fibrin sealant have described internal adhesive applications. This presentation will not be comprehensive, but rather will be an overview to serve as an introduction to this field. Comprehensive reviews of tissue adhesives have been published recently [4–6].

## ACRYLATE ADHESIVES

Several types of clinical usage have been reported for the acrylates. These include wound closure, laceration repair, temporary suspension of soft tissues by applying adhesive to the skin, creation of long-term implants, drug delivery, and endovascular occlusion.

Laceration repair has been reported in several clinical series. The treatment of 1500 children over a period of five years was reported in which cyanoacrylate was used to repair an assortment of superficial skin lacerations in a pediatric emergency room [7]. Among the 1500 patients treated, there were only ten failures and twenty-eight wound infections reported, which is comparable to suture repair. It is unclear, however, how deeply these lacerations penetrated.

In a study of fifty children whose wounds were facial lacerations, it was reported that all were closed with cyanoacrylate adhesive [8]. All of these patients were reported to have superficial lacerations that were less than three centimeters in length. Only five wound complications were reported.

A randomized control trial recently reported a comparison of suture closure and Histoacryl Blue® adhesive for lacerations seen in a pediatric emergency room [9]. This study described superior results utilizing the adhesive in terms of time required to close the wound and the long-term cosmesis.

In each series, the cyanoacrylate was applied to the surface of the wound. When the wound involved the deep dermis, closure was accomplished by deeply placed sutures as an adjunct to the adhesive. In this setting, the application of cyanoacrylate would correspond to the equivalent of a steri-strip.

Closure of the suture line using cyanoacrylate has also been reported in a group of 100 facial-aesthetic surgery patients having a total of 225 wounds. Once again, the subcutaneous layer was often closed with sutures in a separate layer [10]. In a unique application of cyanoacrylate adhesive, twenty patients were randomized to have the surface layer of their episiotomy wound closed with either cyanoacrylate or chromic suture in the skin layer [11]. All of the patients had muscle and deep, soft tissues repaired in layers with chromic sutures according to conventional guidelines. Those patients who had their skin closed by repair with cyanoacrylate reported less pain postoperatively.

Cyanoacrylate has also been used to close skin incisions in groin wounds [12]. Twenty-three patients with groin incisions were studied. The deep dermis was always closed with Dexon®, and the closure of the skin was randomly assigned to either cyanoacrylate, or suture repair with a subcuticular layer of Dexon®. The skin closures with cyanoacrylate were judged to have superior cosmetic results.

One of the recognized hazards of working with cyanoacrylate adhesives is the undesired gluing together of one's fingers when handling the adhesive material. This property of joining normal surfaces of skin to one another was exploited in two different series. The first series described the use of cyanoacrylate to join eyelids and protect corneas in a group of patients who had seventh cranial nerve palsy. This temporary tarsorrhaphy was easily created and lasted for a week at a time [13]. Patients who required several repeat applications would be referred for permanent conventional tarsorrhaphy, since the palsy did not appear to be reversible.

The second report described the use of cyanoacrylate to reposition lower eyelid skin and/or the punctum in order to simulate eyelid surgery for correction of epiphora [14]. This lateral and superior folding of the skin was held in place with cyanoacrylate to give the patient and surgeon a sense of what surgery could accomplish.

Long-term implantation of methyl methacrylate has been reported for use in cranioplasty when adequate bone is unavailable [15]. A recent study reported the creation of a temporary implant substituting for a missing segment of mandible in order to facilitate closure after tumor resection [16]. Tobramycin was mixed into the methyl methacrylate, and it was thought that the antibiotic decreased the risk of infection.

A recent study showed that antibiotics such as gentamycin, which are often admixed into methyl methacrylate during the polymerization process, will be stored in the bubbles that form as the resin sets [17]. The antibiotic will then be released to the surface of the implant through cracks in the resin rather than diffusing through the resin itself.

In a related study, investigators exposed osteoblasts derived from calvarium in tissue culture to gentamycin and to methyl methacrylate monomer [18]. Both of the substances were toxic to bone cells. It was theorized by the authors that the toxicity posed by these two substances may account for some of the loosening observed after bone implants, such as hip prostheses, are placed.

A recent report described a less toxic derivative of cyanoacrylate (polyisohexylcyanoacrylate) [19]. This substance was fabricated in nanoparticle form to be used as a delivery vehicle for doxorubicin, a potent chemotherapeutic with severe toxicity, which was conjugated to the nanoparticles. Binding of the chemotherapeutic agent to the nanoparticles targeted the drug on metastatic implants in lung, liver, and spleen. Particles were trapped in the patients' reticuloendothelial systems, and decreased the toxicity to their hearts and kidneys. The use of cytotoxic cyanoacrylate particles alters the therapeutic index as well as the half life of the drug.

Cyanoacrylate is known to be toxic to the endothelium, a contraindication to its use in closing the deeper layers of the wounds. This property has been exploited by a number of interventional radiologists. A study was done on twenty-nine patients with cerebral arteriovenous malformation who were treated with 2-butyl-*n*-cyanoacrylate [20]. Three of these patients were brought to total occlusion, while several others had partial benefit from the procedure. It was observed that patients with lesions greater than six centimeters in diameter did not derive any benefit from this substance.

A related report noted the successful obliteration with cyanoacrylate of a malformation in the mandible [21]. No recurrence with the use of cyanoacrylate was reported. Not only was there no recurrence of the lesion at four years, but actual replacement of the lesion by normal bone occurred.

## FIBRIN SEALANT

Several types of clinical usages will be described in this report: attachment of skin grafts, closure of wounds, fixation of tissue flaps, securing of subcutaneous implants, control of tissue adhesions, and anastomosis of vessels. In addition, studies are under way to investigate the delivery of various drugs.

Securing skin grafts with fibrin glue continues to be refined. A recent report described the use of autologous fibrin glue to secure the skin grafts on eleven burn patients. A 100% take was reported in nine of the patients and a 90% take reported in the other two [22]. It was the investigators' impression that the fibrin glue facilitated hemostasis as well as adherence of the skin graft and led to the high rate of intake. The study has subsequently been expanded to nineteen patients with seventeen of the nineteen experiencing greater than 90% graft take [23].

A similar study at the University of Virginia reported on the use of single-donor fibrin glue for a series of patients with hand burns [24]. In each case, there was enhanced adherence to the recipient wound bed when grafts were applied with fibrin glue. This series also reported a very high percentage of graft take.

A third study of fibrin glue on hand burns compared quantitatively both motor function and skin sensation [25]. Unfortunately, this study was sequential and not randomized. This report suggested improved function and sensation in burns where the patients had glue applied to secure their skin grafts.

Autologous fibrin adhesive has also been used to secure skin grafts on leg ulcers [26]. In this series one-half of a skin graft was secured on the wound by using sutures, while the other half of the skin graft was secured with fibrin glue. Although no difference was noted in healing, the investigators felt that there was a stronger adherence of the skin graft with the glue. This might have some clinical significance.

Fibrin glue has also been used to facilitate the handling of cultured skin. Cultured human skin keratinocytes are generally prepared on tissue culture plates. Preparation for use in the operating room requires use of the enzyme dispase to interrupt the bridges from the cells to the culture plate. In a recent report [27], standard bacterial culture dishes were coated with fibrin glue and the final plating of cells was performed on this layer rather than on a tissue culture plate. The entire complex of cells and fibrin coating could then be lifted off without the enzyme dispase. The investigators were then able to place the graft onto a patient's wound with the fibrin glue layer on the outer surface away from the wound. The long-term biopsies at one year showed maturation of the skin with formation of anchoring structures. This resembles previous reports of cultured epidermis placed on the wounds. It is possible that this handling of the tissue culture on fibrin glue, without the use of dispase, may enhance the development of anchoring structures from epidermis to the wound bed.

Fibrin glue has also been used to secure full-thickness skin grafts. One study reported on forty patients who were followed for at least four months [28]. Successful take was reported in thirty-nine of the forty patients who had their grafts secured with glue and covered with a very light dressing.

The closure of blepharoplasty wounds has been reported with autologous fibrin glue in a series of thirty-two patients [29]. In this series, only one patient healed with a poor scar. It should be noted that sutures were used to close all deep wound layers, as well as the skin, in the lateral pole of the wound.

Marchac has reported on his use of fibrin glue during a variety of plastic surgical procedures including facelift and abdominoplasty [30]. He demonstrated a decreased need for drains in this series of patients who were treated with commercially available fibrin glue in Europe (Tisseel®). Laboratory studies have been carried out at the University of Virginia using rat models of both radical neck dissection and mastectomy [31,32]. In both cases, the incidence of seroma was decreased in this animal model. It was concluded that there was a decreased need for drain placement in these instances when fibrin glue was used.

The compatibility of the fibrin adhesive with various alloplastic materials was assessed in vivo [33]. No apparent toxicity was noted when comparing placement of implants without fibrin glue. Securing implants in a subcutaneous pocket was thought to be enhanced when fibrin glue was used. This study opens the door for modulation of patient-implant interactions. It is possible that additives to the fibrin glue may be developed to attenuate or enhance the response of a patient to the implant.

Fibrin glue has also been used to facilitate implant handling. Hydroxyapatite granules were mixed with fibrin sealant to create a thick paste that is easy to mold [34]. This paste was used to enhance the contour of the gingiva. The mixture with glue was felt to be more moldable than the paste or powder alone. Fibrin glue has also been used to combine cartilage chips into a moldable implant to increase the availability of local material in rhinoplasty [35]. This innovation decreased the need for harvesting large pieces of cartilage from remote donor sites, such as the ear, thus avoiding the attendant morbidity of graft harvest.

Prevention of adhesion with fibrin glue was reported in a study of flexor tendon injuries in a rabbit model [36]. Fibrin adhesive was compared to suture repair to seal the surface of partial tendon lacerations. Tendons that had been mobilized during the healing phase showed a superior result in those tendons that had been sealed with fibrin glue. This apparent contradiction in the study indicates that the substance used is a two-edged sword and perhaps should be modulated with other additives to prevent adhesion formation. Such modulation could be accomplished theoretically by placing adhesive in a layered configuration. The standard fibrin glue could be placed directly against the suture line and a layer of modified glue placed into the synovial space to inhibit interaction between the tendon and synovial sheath.

Anastomosis of blood vessels has been reported [37]. The problem of the vessel patency was addressed by using polyethylene glycol 4000 to make a moldable, intraluminal stent to keep the vessel open until the anastomosis was complete. Once the anastomosis was complete, reperfusion caused the implant to melt and flush away with the onrush of the blood. This study described the use of two stay sutures, so it was not a completely sutureless anastomosis. A 100% patency rate was reported.

A different approach was reported where the fibrin was blended with indocyanine green dye to enhance its absorption of diode laser light at a near-infrared wavelength [38]. The dye facilitated absorption of energy from the laser onto tissue. This absorbance of energy was thought to enhance the strength of the adhesive bond that the glue produced, while decreasing the damage of the diode light to the adjacent vessel wall. The combination of fibrinogen and dye was described by the authors as a "solder."

Future prospects of fibrin glue as a drug delivery agent include the ability to exploit the presence of fibronectin in the fibrin glue as a substrate that facilitates migration of fibroblasts into the wound. Addition of steroid to fibrin glue might be used to diminish the recurrence of keloid after excision in sealed wounds. Hyaluronic acid might be used to diminish adhesion formation and, similarly, peptide growth factors, such as FGF which is known to accelerate angiogenesis. This might be used to stimulate healing in slow-healing wounds. The agent TFG-$\beta$, which has a demonstrated role in wound healing and scar formation, might be used in its various isoforms to alter wound healing and induce a fetal wound healing state.

Osteoblasts combined with fibrin glue might be injected into bone fracture with or without bone matrix protein. The adipocyte, which is a fastidious cell, might be induced to survive after transplantation from liposuction if it were mixed with fibrin glue and appropriate regulatory peptides, thus replacing alloplastic implants for soft tissue augmentation. Likewise in the case of refractory hernia, biodegradable mesh might be cultured with fibroblasts in such a way that the co-implant might develop into a replacement for missing fascia. In addition, fibrin glue might be used as a reinforcing agent for closure of large wounds that have large, dead, space wounds with tissue flaps. It also might find usage in diminishing the formation of hematoma after liposuction by direct injection into regions that have been treated.

Finally, the development of endoscopic techniques, such as browlift and facelift, might be enhanced by coating wound surfaces with endoscopically applied fibrin glue to diminish the formation of hematoma. Recent developments in cyanoacrylate technology might allow placement of this more powerful adhesive (once it has been rendered more biocompatible) into the wounds to facilitate resuspension of soft tissue.

In summary, the burgeoning data suggest that various components that take part in wound healing, which have previously been identified and characterized, may be used to enhance or diminish wound healing as desired. Thus, fibrin glue can be viewed as a delivery vehicle for these various substances, allowing the design of wound outcomes by actively modulating wound healing.

## REFERENCES

1. Vobel, A., O'Grady, K., Toriumi, D. M. Surgical tissue adhesives in facial, plastic and reconstructive surgery. *Fac. Plast. Surg.*, 9:49–57, 1993.
2. Sierra, D. H. Fibrin sealant adhesive systems: A review of their chemistry, material properties and clinical applications. *J. Biomater. Appl.*, 7:309–352, 1993.
3. Ellis, D. A., Shaikh, A. The ideal tissue adhesive in facial plastic and reconstructive surgery. *J. Otolaryngol.*, 19:68–72, 1990.
4. Lerner, R., Binur, N. S. Current status of surgical adhesives. *J. Surg. Res.*, 48:165–181, 1990.
5. Papatheofanis, F. J., Barmada, R. The principles and applications of surgical adhesives. *Surg. Ann.*, 25(Pt. 1):49–81, 1993.
6. Himel, H. N., Persing, J. A. Tissue adhesives in plastic surgery. In: *Advances in Plastic and Reconstructive Surgery.* 10th ed. Mosby-Year Book, Inc., M. Habal, ed. Chicago. pp. 73–92, 1994.
7. Mizrahi, S., Bickel, A., Ben-Layish, E. Use of tissue adhesive in the repair of lacerations in children. *J. Ped. Surg.*, 23:312–313, 1988.
8. Watson, D. P. Use of cyanoacrylate tissue adhesive for closing facial lacerations in children. *J. Ped. Surg.*, 23:312–313, 1988.
9. Quinn, J. V., Drzewiecki, A., Li, M. M., et al. A randomized, controlled trial comparing a tissue adhesive with suturing in the repair of pediatric facial lacerations. *Ann. Emerg. Med.*, 22:1130–1135, 1993.
10. Kamer, F. M., Joseph, J. H. Histoacryl—its use in aesthetic facial plastic surgery. *Arch. of Otolaryngol. Head Neck Surg.*, 115:193–197, 1989.
11. Adoni, A., Anteby, E. The use of Histoacryl for episiotomy repair. *Br. J. Obstet. Gyn.*, 98:476–478, 1991.
12. Keng, T. M., Bucknall, T. E. A clinical trial of tissue adhesive (Histoacryl) in skin closure of groin wounds. *Med. J. Malaysia,* 44:122–128, 1989.
13. Diamond, J. P. Temporary tarsorraphy with cyanoacrylate adhesive for seventh-nerve palsy [letter]. *The Lancet,* 335:1039, 1990.
14. Khan, J. A. Cyanoacrylate-assisted trial eyelid repositioning for epiphora. *Ophthal. Plast. Reconstr. Surg.*, 7:138–140, 1991.
15. Persing, J. A. Cronin, A. J., Delashaw, J. B., Edgerton, M. T., Henson, S. L.,

Jane, J. A. Late surgical treatment of unilateral coronal synostosis using methyl methacrylate. *J. Neurosurg.*, 66:793–799, 1987.

16. Goode, R. L., Reynolds, B. N. Tobramycin impregnated methylmethacrylate for mandible reconstruction. *Arch. Otolaryngol. Head Neck Surg.*, 118:210, 1992.
17. Baker, A. S., Greenham, L. W. Release of gentamycin from acrylic bone cement. *J. B. J. S.*, 70A:1551–1557, 1988.
18. Pedersen, J. G., Lund, B. Effects of gentamycin and monomer on bone: An in vitro study. *J. Arthroplasty*, 1988.
19. Kattan, J., Droz, J. P., Couvreur, P., et al. Phase I clinical trial and pharmacokinetic evaluation of doxorubicin carried by polyisohexycyanoacrylate nanoparticles. *Invest. New Drugs*, 10:191–199, 1992.
20. Berthelsen, B., Lofgren, J., Svendsen, P. Embolization of cerebral arteriovenous malformations with bucrylate. Experience in a first series of twenty-nine patients. *Acta Radiologica*, 21:12–21, 1990.
21. Shultz, R. E., Richardson, D. D., Kempf, K. K., Pevsner, P. H., George, E. D. Treatment of a central arteriovenous malformation of the mandible with cyanoacrylate: A four-year follow-up. *Oral Surg. Med. Oral Path.*, 65:267–271, 1988.
22. Saltz, R., Dimick, A., Harris, C., Grotting, J. C., Psillakis, J., Vasconez, L. O. Application of autologous fibrin glue in burn wounds. *J. Burn Care Rehab.*, 10:504–507, 1989.
23. Saltz, R., Sierra, D., Feldman, D. S., Saltz, M. B., Dimick, A. Vasconez, L. O. Experimental and clinical applications of fibrin glue [see comments]. *Plast. Reconstr. Surg.*, 88:1005–1015, 1991.
24. Stuart, J. D., Morgan, R. F., Kenney, J. G. Single-donor fibrin glue for hand burns. *Ann. Plast. Surg.*, 24:524–527, 1990.
25. Boeckx, W., Vandevoort, M., Blondeel, P., Van Raemdonck, D., Vandekerckhove, E. Fibrin glue in the treatment of dorsal hand burns. *Burns*, 18:395–400, 1992.
26. Dahlstrom, K. K., Weis-Fogh, U. S., Medgyesi, S., Rostgaard, J., Sorensen, H. The use of autologous fibrin adhesive in skin transplantation [see comments]. *Plast. Reconstr. Surg.*, 90:968–972, 1992.
27. Ronfard, V., Broly, H., Mitchell, V., et al. Use of human keratinocytes cultured on fibrin glue in the treatment of burn wounds. *Burns*, 17:181–194, 1991.
28. Chakravorty, R. C., Sosnowski, K. M. Autologous fibrin glue in full-thickness skin grafting. *Ann. Plast. Surg.*, 21:488–491, 1989.
29. Mandel, M. A. Minimal suture blepharoplasty: Closure of incisions with autologous fibrin glue. *Aesth. Plast. Surg.*, 16:269–272, 1992.
30. Marchac, D., Pugash, E., Gault, D. The use of sprayed fibrin glue for facelifts. *Eur. J. Plast. Surg.*, 10:139–143, 1987.
31. Lindsey, W. H., Masterson, T. M., Llaneras, M., Spotnitz, W. D., Wanebo, H. J., Morgan, R. F. Seroma prevention using fibrin glue during modified radical neck dissection in a rat model. *Amer. J. Surg.*, 156:310–313, 1988.
32. Lindsey, W. H., Masterson, T. M., Spotnitz, W. D., Wilhelm, M. C., Morgan, R. F. Seroma prevention using fibrin glue in a rat mastectomy model. *Arch. Surg.*, 125:305–307, 1990.

33. Feldman, M., Sataloff, R. T., Choi, H. Y., Ballas, S. K. Compatibility of autologous fibrin adhesive with implant materials. *Arch. Otolaryngol. Head Neck Surg.*, 114:182–185, 1988.
34. Wittkampf, A. R. Fibrin glue as cement for HA-granules. *J. Cran. Maxillo. Fac. Surg.*, 17:179–181, 1989.
35. Fontana, A., Muti, E., Cicerale, D., Rizzotti, M. Cartilage chips synthesized with fibrin glue in rhinoplasty. *Aesth. Plast. Surg.*, 15:237–240, 1991.
36. Frykman, E., Jacobsson, S., Widenfalk, B. Fibrin sealant in prevention of flexor tendon adhesions: An experimental study in the rabbit. *J. Hand Surg.*, 18A:68–75, 1993.
37. Kamiji, T., Maeda, M., Matsumoto, K., Nishioka, K. Microvascular anastomosis using polyethylene glycol 4000 and fibrin glue. *Br. J. Plast. Surg.*, 42:54–58, 1989.
38. Oz, M. C., Johnson, J. P., Parangi, S., et al. Tissue soldering by use of indocyanine green dye-enhanced fibrinogen with the near infrared diode laser. *J. Vasc. Surg.*, 11:718–725, 1990.

# *Chapter 20: Clinical Applications of Tissue Adhesives in Aesthetic and Reconstructive Surgery*[1]

R. SALTZ

## INTRODUCTION

Throughout the centuries, surgeons and scientists have sought an ideal surgical sealant and adhesive, one that would be safe, biologically compatible, with rapid action and adequate tensile strength. This long history goes back to 1100 B.C., when Egyptian technology had developed a variety of adhesives, including gum from acacia trees and several types of resin.

Sutures are still the most common technique for closure of wounds. However, in this century, significant progress was observed in the development of surgical biological adhesives. From Bergel [1] to the most recent European experience [2–8], the clinical application of tissue glues in the surgical arena has increased significantly.

This chapter presents some of the clinical applications of surgical adhesives in the management of skin grafts in burn patients, in difficult wounds, and innovations in the application of tissue glues when combined with aesthetic and endoscopic surgery. The emphasis is placed on the aesthetic considerations in facial burns, hand burns, and facial surgery. This large clinical experience has been accomplished utilizing autologous fibrin glue or single-donor fibrin glue obtained by the cryoprecipitate method [9–12].

## FUNCTIONAL AND AESTHETIC RECONSTRUCTION OF BURNED HANDS

There is still significant controversy concerning the management of deep, partial-thickness burns to the hands. Treatment alternatives for dorsal burns

[1]Portions of this chapter are reproduced from References [11] and [12] with permission.

include early excision and grafting, topical enzymes and agents with grafting if necessary. Long-term follow-up studies compare different types of treatments of burned hands, but the same physical therapy, splinting, and scar compression techniques have failed to demonstrate significant differences in the functional results [13].

Most of the studies failed to address the aesthetic aspects of the reconstruction of the burned hands. Grafting with sheet grafts seems to offer the best aesthetic results yet. We have used fibrin glue to secure sheet grafts with excellent results [11,12]. In an attempt to obtain a better aesthetic result in burned hands, sheet grafts secured with fibrin glue were used.

Intravenous resuscitation and topical treatments with Silvadene® were done for the first twenty-four to forty-eight hours. After an accurate estimate of burn depth, definitive surgical care was begun. Under general anesthesia and tourniquet control to minimize blood loss, the burned hands were debrided down to viable tissue. After adequate hemostasis, medium split thickness of skin grafts (0.012–0.016 in), appropriately tailored to the burned extremity, were secured in place with autologous or single-donor fibrin glue. Only a few stay sutures were necessary. Xeroform dressing was used as a light dressing and the hands immobilized in a splint for twenty-four hours. Passive and active motion was started as early as the second postoperative day. Compression garments were started at twenty-one days.

Graft take was over 96% in our series. All patients were able to start early active and passive motion with an excellent functional and aesthetic result in long-term follow-ups. The biological adhesive decreases bleeding during the procedure due to its hemostatic effect, secures the graft in place, and avoids hematoma formation that often results in graft loss. This makes possible the use of sheets instead of meshed grafts. When compared with conventional treatment in our own patients, this technique offers a shorter hospital stay for isolated burns to the hands, minimal postoperative care and immobilization, no pressure dressings, prompt start of physical therapy with an early return to normal activities, and a definitively better aesthetic appearance. The combination of fibrin glue and sheet grafts seems to be the ideal treatment for burned hands (Figures 20.1 and 20.2).

## AESTHETIC RECONSTRUCTION OF FACIAL BURNS

Excision and immediate grafting early after burn injury has gained increasing acceptance in the management of burns to the face. It provides several advantages: a decrease in duration, of convalescence time, and in the total number of anesthetics needed [14,15].

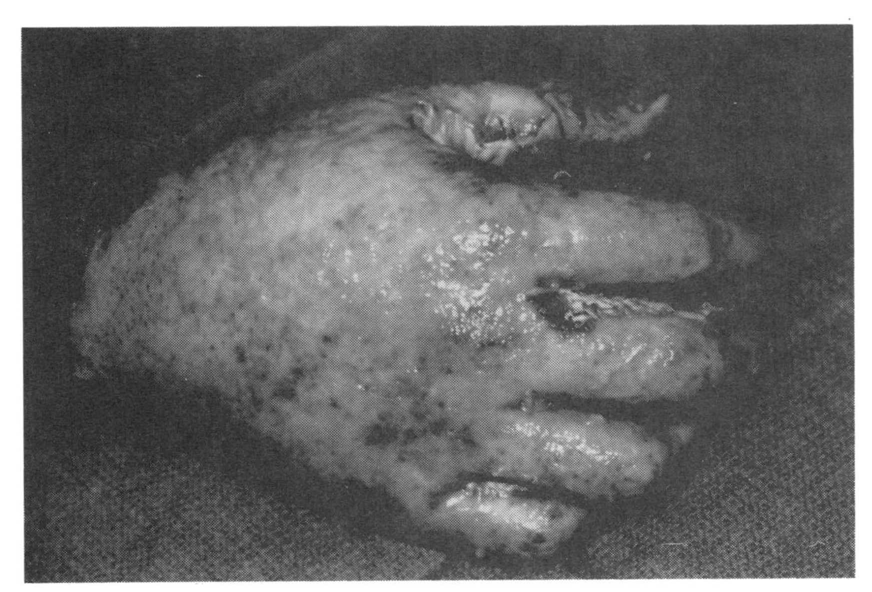

**FIGURE 20.1a**
Deep second- and third-degree burns to right hand.

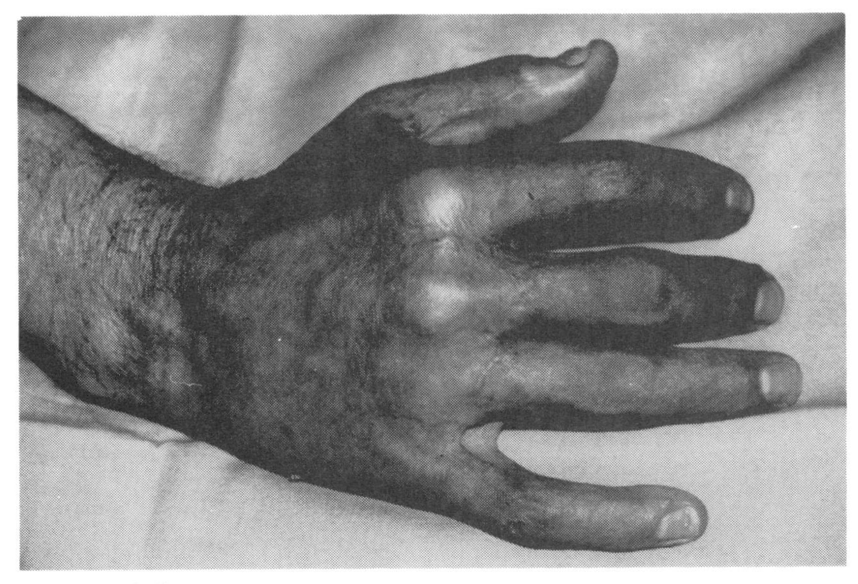

**FIGURE 20.1b**
Three-month postoperative view. Excellent range of motion and aesthetic appearance.

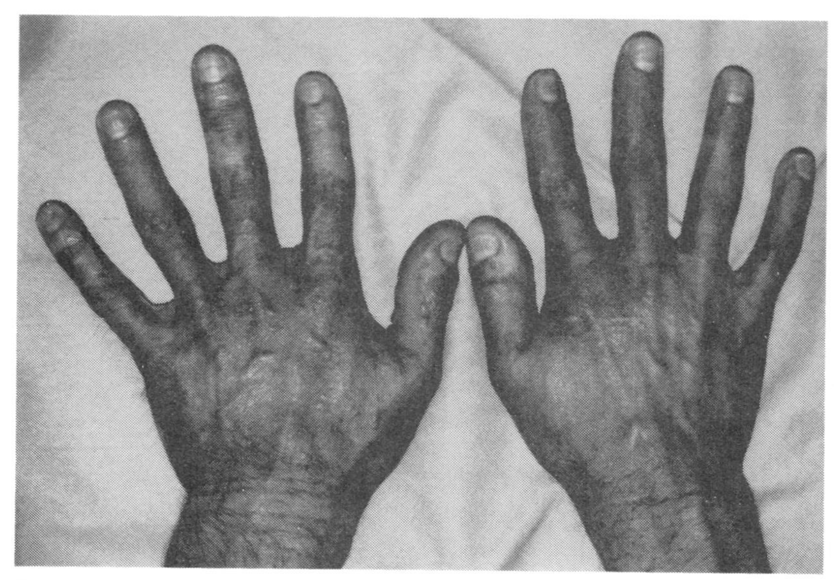

**FIGURE 20.2a**
Deep second- and third-degree burns to both hands. Reconstruction performed with sheet grafts and fibrin glue.

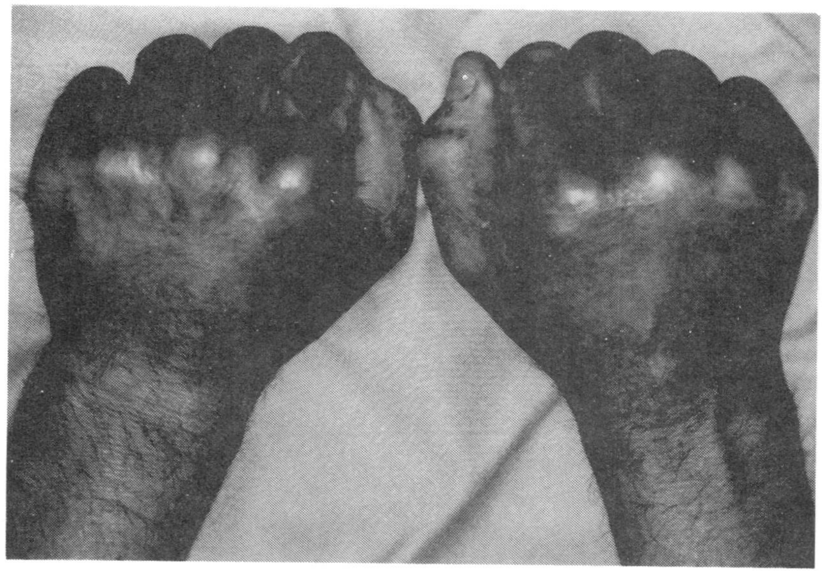

**FIGURE 20.2b**
Excellent range of motion and aesthetic appearance.

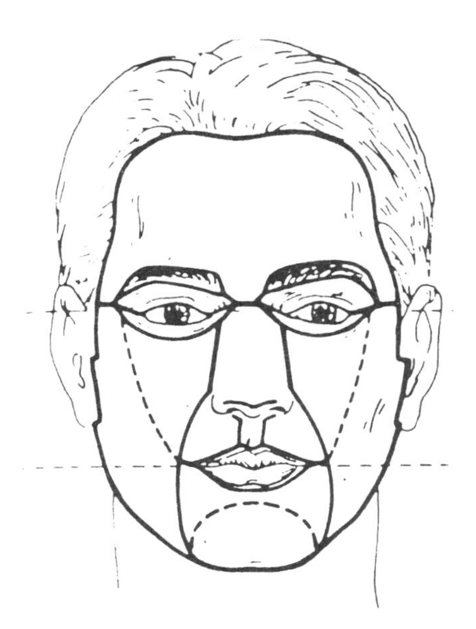

**FIGURE 20.3a**
Facial aesthetic units.

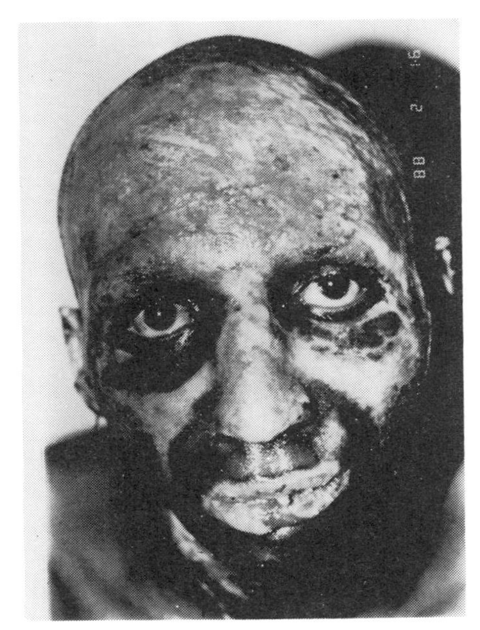

**FIGURE 20.3b**
Third-degree burn to forehead.

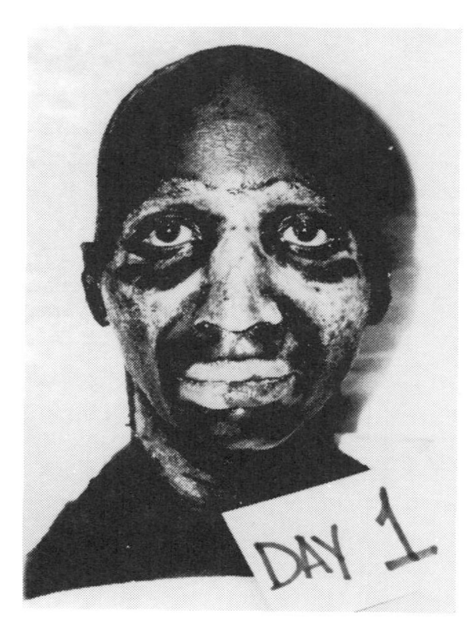


**FIGURE 20.3c**
Facial aesthetic unit resurfaced with sheet graft secured only with fibrin glue.

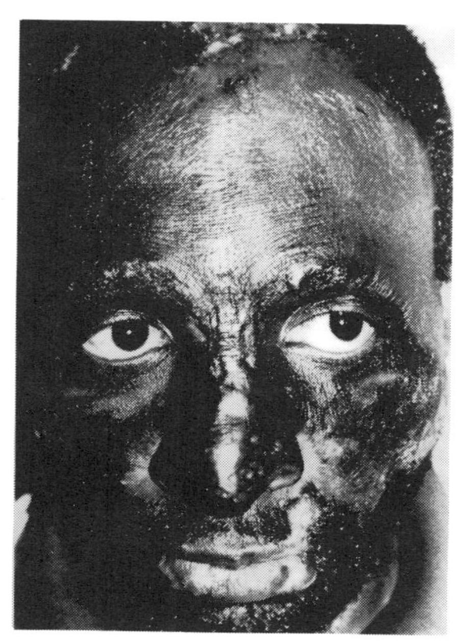

**FIGURE 20.3d**
Long-term appearance.

Resurfacing of facial burns with sheet grafts demands significant and prolonged postoperative care and results in a suboptimal graft take. To obtain better function and appearance, minimal blood loss, and increased graft survival with minimal postoperative care, deep facial burns were treated by sequential excision and grafting with the grafts secured with AFG in one single operation.

Five significant advantages in using fibrin adhesive to difficult recipient sites have been documented [3]. Ihara and Stuart [16,17] have shown that the hemostatic effect in fixation of skin grafts was augmented with the use of fibrin glue. They have also shown reduced blood transfusions, reduced operative time, and reduced lengths of stay in the hospital for those patients.

Facial burns that were not healed at ten days [15] were tangentially excised down to viable tissue and immediately grafted with medium-thickness skin sheet grafts. These grafts were secured in place with autologous fibrin glue in accordance with the aesthetic units of the face. These grafts were obtained from the most suitable donor site available with an appropriate match in color and texture.

Gentle, uniform pressure was applied over the entire unit for two to three minutes immediately after the glue was placed. A Xeroform dressing was used to cover the whole aesthetic unit. Donor sites were also covered with Xeroform dressings (Sherwood Medical, St. Louis, MO). The units were

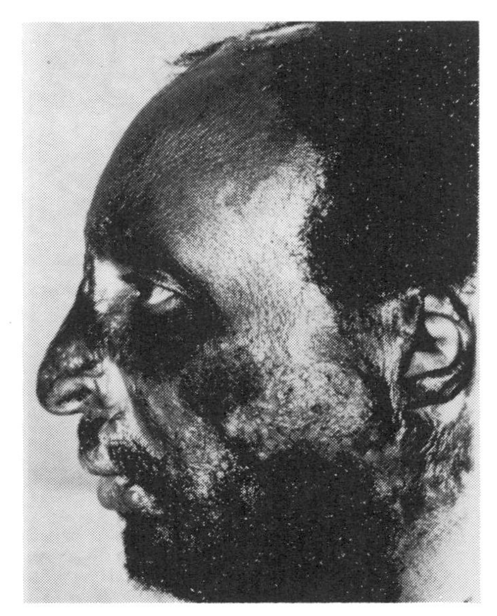

**FIGURE 20.3e**
Long-term appearance.

then inspected for any fluid collections, which were aspirated with an insulin syringe.

The graft take was 100% and the aesthetic result was very satisfactory. The patients were able to move, eat and ambulate on the first postoperative day. Color and texture matches have been very satisfactory in treated patients, who now have been followed up for several years (Figure 20.3).

## GRAFTING WOUNDS AT DIFFICULT SITES

Fibrin glue was used to improve the early adherence of skin grafts to wounds at difficult sites [11]. This, otherwise, would have required bolster-type dressings and long-term immobilization. These wounds were on the scalp, neck, shoulder, back, buttocks, hands, and legs. Again, graft survival above 90% was observed in this population. Minimal postoperative care was required and some of these patients were treated on out-patient basis (Figures 20.4 and 20.5).

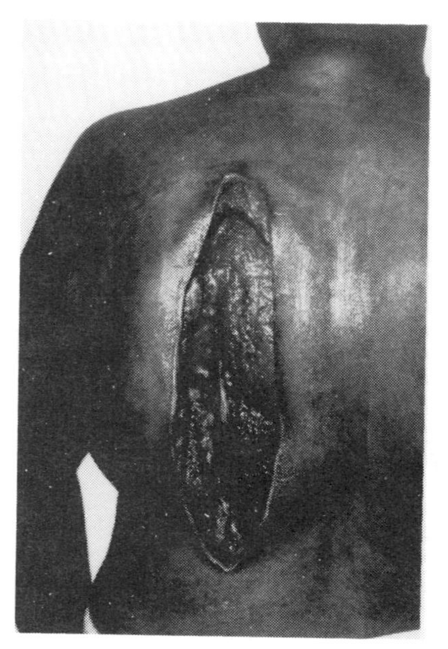

**FIGURE 20.4a**
Diabetic elderly patient who developed necrotizing fascitis and required extensive debridement.

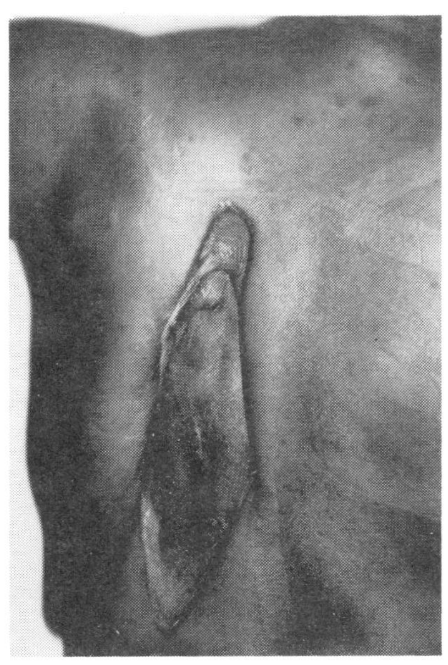

**FIGURE 20.4b**
Wound completely resurfaced with split-thickness skin graft secured only with fibrin glue, no dressings were necessary. The patient was out of bed and fully ambulatory on the second postoperative day.

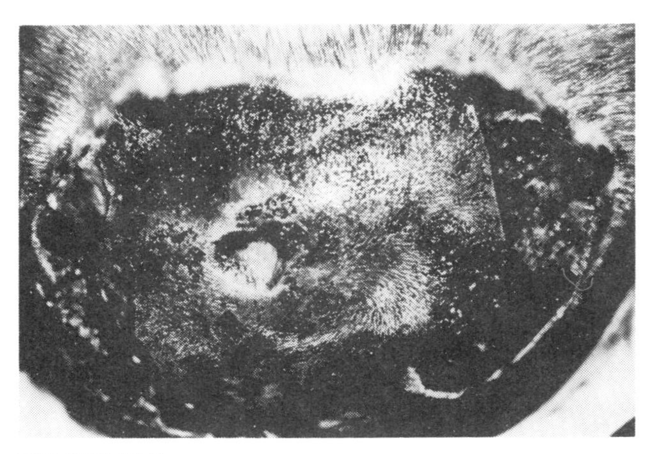

**FIGURE 20.5a**
High-voltage electrical burns to scalp.

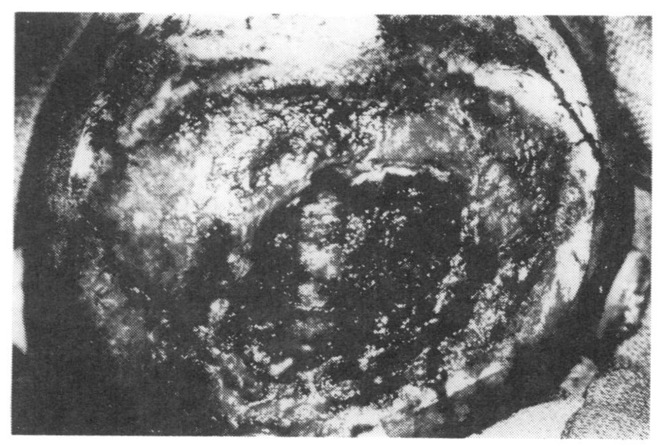

**FIGURE 20.5b**
Extensive debridement that involved necrotic soft tissues and bone.

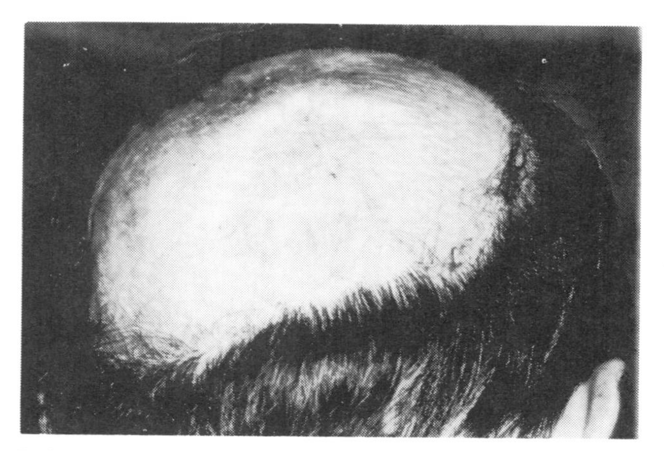

**FIGURE 20.5c**
Complete resurfacing of burned scalp with skin graft secured only with fibrin glue.

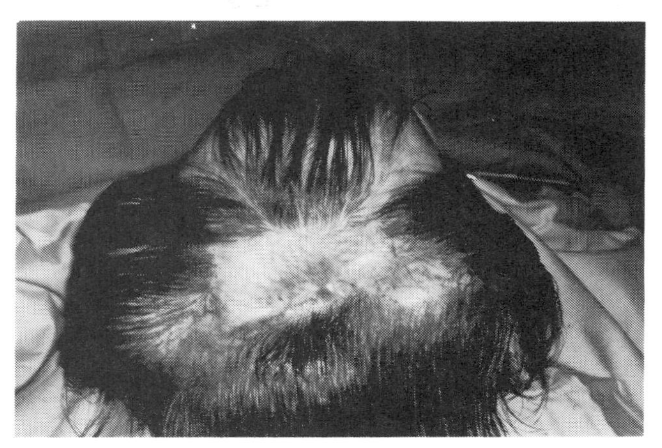

**FIGURE 20.5d**
Tissue expansion for reconstruction of burn alopecia.

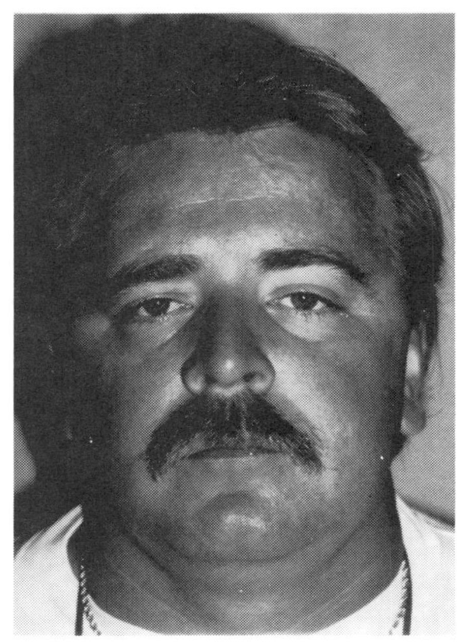

**FIGURE 20.5e**
Result.

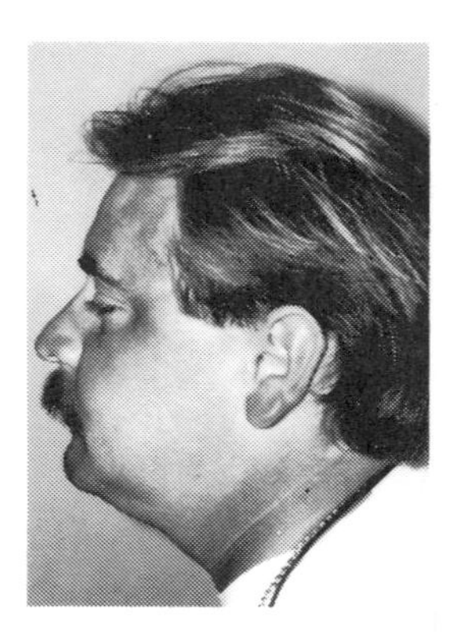

**FIGURE 20.5f**
Result.

## TISSUE ADHESIVES AND AESTHETIC SURGERY

Several advantages have been documented in the use of tissue adhesives in aesthetic surgery. The European experience has shown that tissue glues have decreased the incidence of hematoma formation and edema, avoid painful suture removal, and, in some cases, help to obtain an earlier, pleasant result in facial aesthetic surgical cases [7]. Marchac has described its use as a substitution for sutures in rhytidectomies and blepharoplasties [8]. Unlike the European experience, in the United States only autologous fibrin glue has been used in aesthetic patients for these elective procedures. The FDA has not yet approved the commercial pool-donor glue for fear of any potential risks of viral transmission (Figure 20.6).

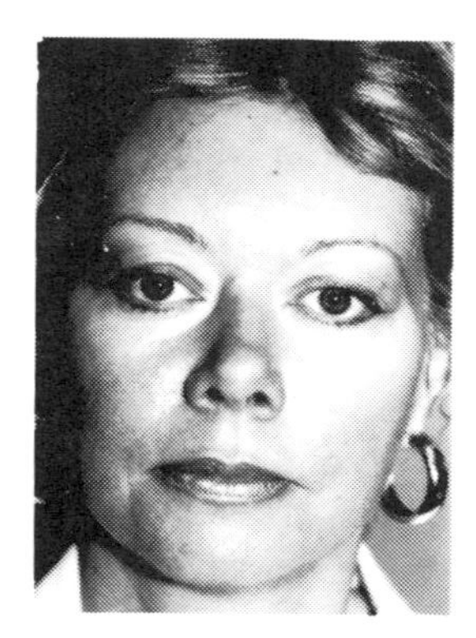

**FIGURE 20.6a**
Preoperative view.

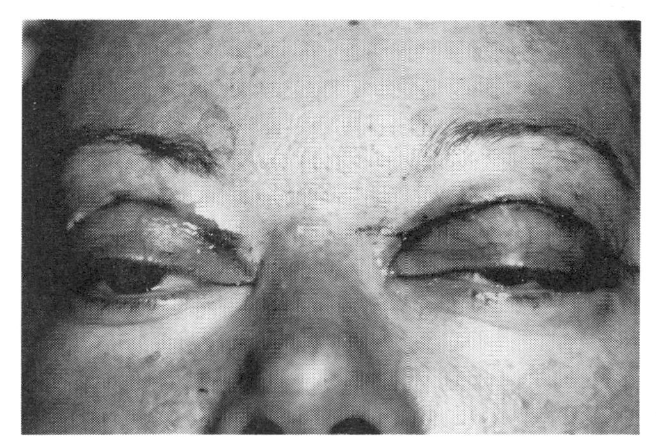

**FIGURE 20.6b**
Blepharoplasty. Right side closed with sutures. Left side closed with autologous fibrin glue.

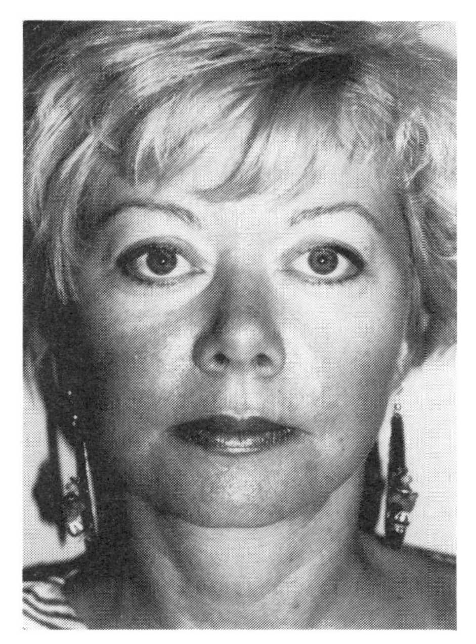

**FIGURE 20.6c**
Postoperative view.

## TISSUE ADHESIVES AND ENDOSCOPIC SURGERY

Endoscopic surgery has become a popular procedure among all surgical specialties. Surgeons around the world have taken advantage of this new technology to obtain good and safe results with smaller scars and less morbidity. Plastic surgeons for the last three years have taken this new technology to new dimensions [18–21]. The goal in aesthetic surgery is to create beauty and balance, while minimizing evidence of the surgical approach. Endoscopic surgery is now being applied to browlifting and facelifting by avoiding a coronal incision, thus minimizing morbidity.

One of the controversial aspects in endo-browlift continues to be the ideal method of fixation. Several authors describe different approaches that involve sutures, miniscrews, and external dressings [18–24]. I have used autologous tissue glue as a method of fixation and the preliminary results have been very satisfactory. The adhesive not only helps to secure the forehead and scalp flaps in place, but also works as a hemostatic agent, decreasing hematoma formation and bruising. A combination of injection of tissue adhesive at the end of the procedure and application of a light pressure dressing seems to be, in this preliminary experience, an excellent method for fixation after endoscopic browlift. This technique will probably be limited to younger patients who do not have significant amounts of excess skin, where a more invasive technique of fixation would be recommended. Marchac [25] has also observed these advantages in the use of tissue adhesives in endoscopic aesthetic surgery (Figure 20.7).

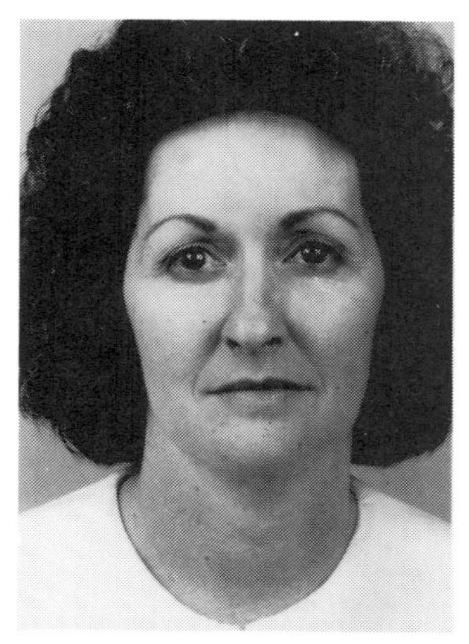

**FIGURE 20.7a**
Preoperative view.

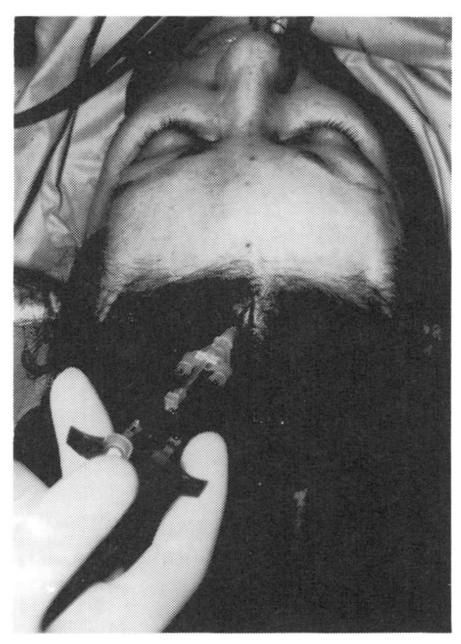

**FIGURE 20.7b**
Endoscopic browlift and facelift. Fibrin glue used to help with hemostasis and secure tissues, thus avoiding sutures.

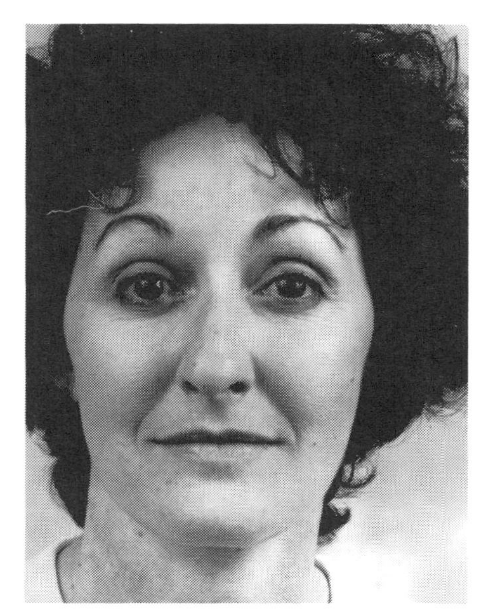

**FIGURE 20.7c**
Postoperative view.

## ACKNOWLEDGEMENT

The author wishes to thank Ms. Andrea Reeder for assistance with this chapter.

## REFERENCES

1. Bergel, S. Uber wirkungen des fibrins. *Dtsch. Med. Wochenschr.*, 35:663, 1909.
2. Matras, H. Fibrin seal: The state of the art. *J. Oral Maxillofac. Surg.*, 43:605, 1985.
3. Vibe, P., Pless, J. A new method of skin graft adhesion. *Scand. J. Plast. Reconstr. Surg.*, 17:263, 1983.
4. Spangler, H. P., Holle, J., Braun, F., et al. Die verklebung experimenteller leberverletzungenmittels hochkonzentriertem fibrin. *Acta Chir. Austriaca*, 7:89, 1975.
5. Spangler, H. P., Holle, J., Braun, F. Gewebeklebung mit fibrin: Eine experimentelle studie an der rattenhaut. *Wien. Klin. Wochenschr.*, 85:827, 1973.
6. Kletter, G., Matras, H., Dinges, H. P. Zur paratiellen klebung von mikrogefass-anastomosen im intrakraniellen bereich. *Wien. Klin. Wochenschr.*, 90:415, 1978.
7. Bruck, H. G. Fibrin tissue adhesion and its use in rhytidectomy: A pilot study. *Aesthetic Plast. Surg.*, 6:197, 1982.
8. Marchac, D., Pugash, E., Gault, D. The use of sprayed fibrin glue for facelifts. *Eur. J. Plast. Surg.*, 10:139, 1987.
9. Dresdale, A., Rose, E. A., Jeevanandum, V., et al. Preparation of fibrin glue from single-donor fresh-frozen plasma. *Surgery*, 97:750, 1985.
10. Spotnitz, W. D., Mintz, P. D., Avery, N., et al. Fibrin glue from stored human plasma: An inexpensive and efficient method for local blood bank preparation. *Ann. Surg.*, 53:460, 1987.
11. Saltz, R., Dimick, A., Harris, C., et al. Application of autologous fibrin glue in burn wounds. *J. Burn Care Rehabil.*, 10:504, 1989.
12. Saltz, R., Sierra, D., Feldman, D., et al. Experimental and clinical applications of fibrin glue. *Plast. Reconstr. Surg.*, 88:6, 1991.
13. Salisbury, R. E., Wright, P. Evaluation of early excision of dorsal burns of the hand. *Plast. Reconstr. Surg.*, 69(4):670, 1987.
14. Janzekovic, Z. A new concept in the early excision and immediate grafting of burns. *J. Trauma*, 10:1103, 1970.
15. Engrav, L. H., Heimbach, D. M., Walkinshaw, M. D., et al. Excision of burns of the face. *Plast. Reconstr. Surg.*, 77:744–751, 1986.
16. Ihara, N. et al. Application of fibrin glue to burns: Its hemostatic and transplant fixation effects in the excised wounds. *Burns Incl. Therm. Inj.*, 10:396, 1984.
17. Stuart, J. D., Kenney, J. G., Lettieri, J., et al. Application of single-donor fibrin glue to burns. *J. Burn Care Rehabil.*, 9:619–622, 1988.
18. Core, G. B., Vasconez, L. O., Askren, C., et al. Coronal facelift with endoscopic techniques. *Plast. Surg. Forum*, 15:227, 1992.

19. Saltz, R., Stowers, R., Smith, M., et al. Laparoscopically harvested omental free flap to cover a soft tissue defect. *Ann. Surg.*, 217:542–547, 1993.
20. Rosenberg, P., Miller, M., Saltz, R., et al. Laparoscopic harvest of the jejunum for esophageal reconstruction. *Plast. Surg. Forum,* 16:267–268, 1993.
21. Price, C. I., Eaves, III, F. F., Nahai, F., et al. Endoscopic transaxillary subpectoral breast augmentation. *Plast. Reconstr. Surg.*, 94:612–619, 1994.
22. Ramirez, O. M. Endoscopic techniques in facial rejuvenation: An overview. *Aesth. Plast. Surg.*, 18:141, 1994.
23. Isse, N. Personal communication–Endoscopy in Plastic Surgery: A Multidisciplinary Symposium. Birmingham, AL, July, 1994.
24. Daniels, R. Personal communication–Endoscopy in Plastic Surgery: A Multidisciplinary Symposium. Birmingham, AL, July, 1994.
25. Marchac, D. Personal communication–European Association of Plastic Surgeons. Geneva, May, 1994.

# *Chapter 21: Surgical Adhesives in Otolaryngology*

K. H. SIEDENTOP

The criteria for an ideal tissue adhesive are that it:

(1) May be used on moist tissues
(2) Distributes evenly over the tissue surface
(3) Forms a durable bond in a few seconds between the tissues to be united
(4) Does not cause tissue damage locally or generally
(5) Is not carcinogenic
(6) Biodegrades in a relatively short period of time

In the past, three different cyanoacrylates were used as tissue adhesives for diverse surgical problems. Two of these, isobutyl-cyanoacrylate and methyl-methacrylate, create severe inflammation and tissue destruction in the middle and inner ear of dogs, guinea pigs, and cats; therefore, these two adhesives were considered unsuitable. The adhesive 2-butyl-cyano-acrylate or Histoacryl®, which seemed to come closest to the requirements for an ideal tissue glue, was tested in the early 1970s.

In middle-ear surgery on twenty dog ears, Histoacryl® was used in the experimental ear, while in the opposite control ear, the identical operation was performed without glue. Structures united with tissue adhesive were: (1) fascia graft to tympanic membrane; (2) cartilage strut to stapes footplate; (3) bone strut to footplate; (4) incus interposition between malleus and stapes (Figures 21.1 and 21.2).

These experiments indicated that Histoacryl®, when used in small amounts, was not damaging to middle- and inner-ear structures, and biodegraded within a limited period of time, creating a stable tissue union.

To further evaluate the possible effects of using Histoacryl® in the human middle and inner ear, this adhesive was experimentally applied to the oval window and stapes region of nine baboon middle ears. In most of the animals

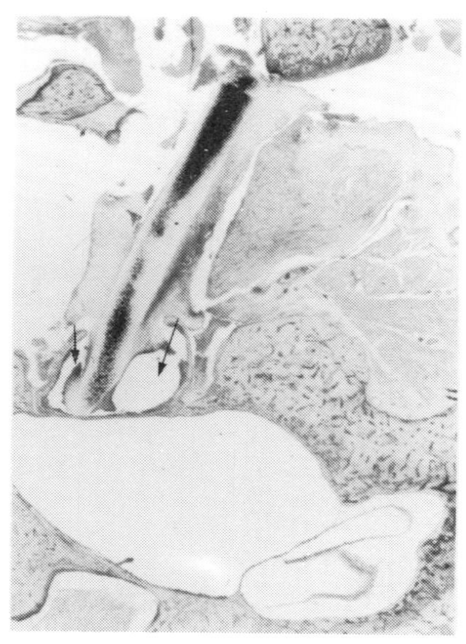

**FIGURE 21.1**
The oval window region of a large dog. A cartilage strut was glued to the middle-ear surface of the stapes footplate. Footplate and labyrinth structures are intact. Arrows indicate the washed-out glue bubble.

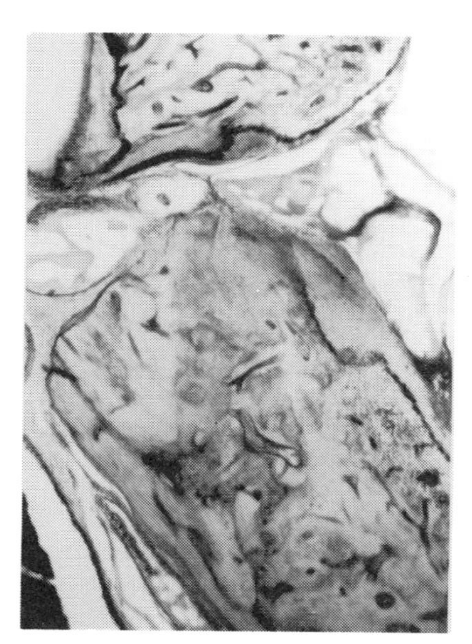

**FIGURE 21.2**
Incus interposition reveals good adherence of bone to bone.

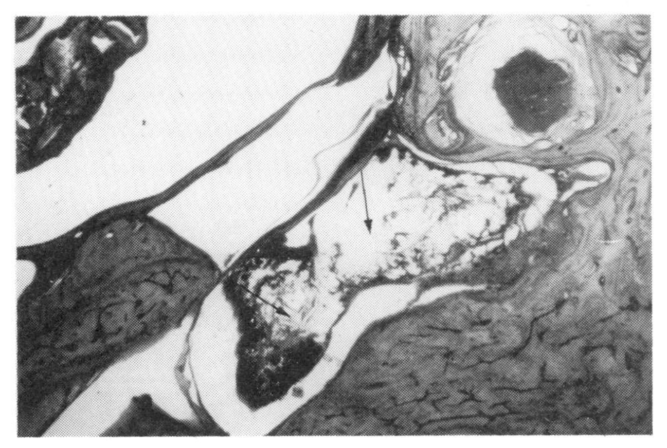

**FIGURE 21.3**
Tissue adhesive fills the entire recess between oval window and round window. Round window membrane is intact. Arrows indicate the adhesive bubble.

the adhesive filled the entire recess between the oval window and round window. Histologic sections of this region revealed the round window membrane, stapes footplate, labyrinth, and middle ear did not show any damage or injury due to the adhesive applications. Only minor inflammatory reactions were observed to surround the adhesive bubbles (Figures 21.3 and 21.4).

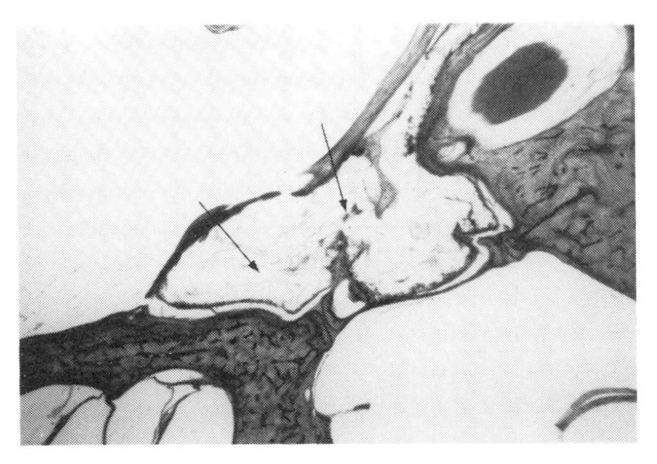

**FIGURE 21.4**
Oval window region of another baboon's ear. Adhesive is seen filling the area between promontory and facial nerve. Stapes crura are broken away. Footplate and labyrinth structures are intact. Arrows point to the large adhesive bubble.

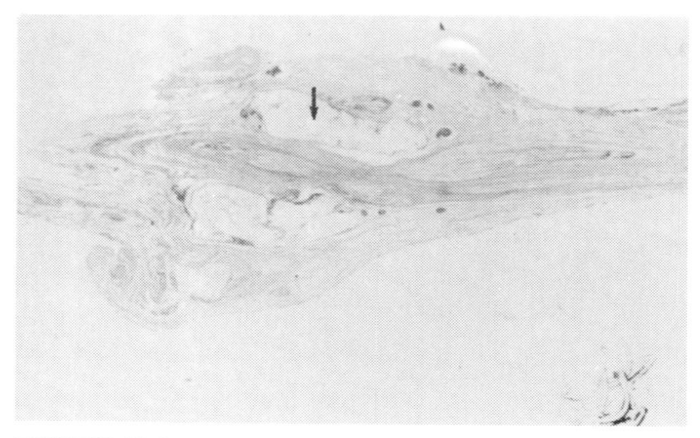

**FIGURE 21.5**
Facial nerve repaired with sutures through neurilemma and silastic collar. Nerve fibers continue through repair site. Arrow points to silastic collar.

In another experiment, Histoacryl® was tested on facial nerve repairs of dogs. Thirteen nerves were repaired: seven with Histoacryl® and six with sutures and a silastic sheath. Success was judged on two criteria: (1) observation of motion in the muscles that were innervated after electrical stimulation of the nerve proximal to the repair site; (2) evaluation of microanatomical continuity. The two repair methods produced statistically equal results (Figures 21.5, 21.6, 21.7 and 21.8).

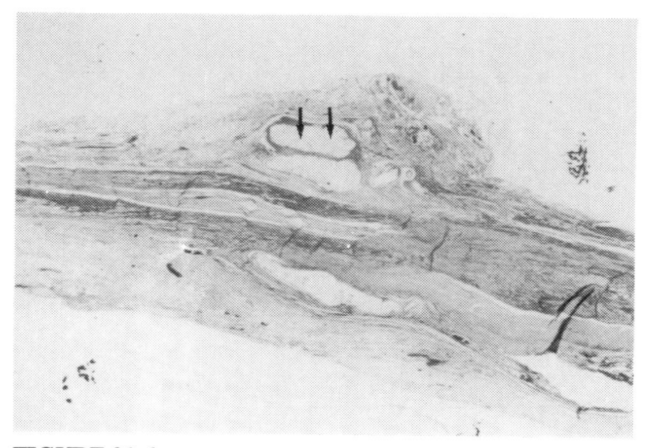

**FIGURE 21.6**
Facial nerve repair with tissue adhesive collar. Nerve fibers continue through repair site. Arrow points to small adhesive bubble.

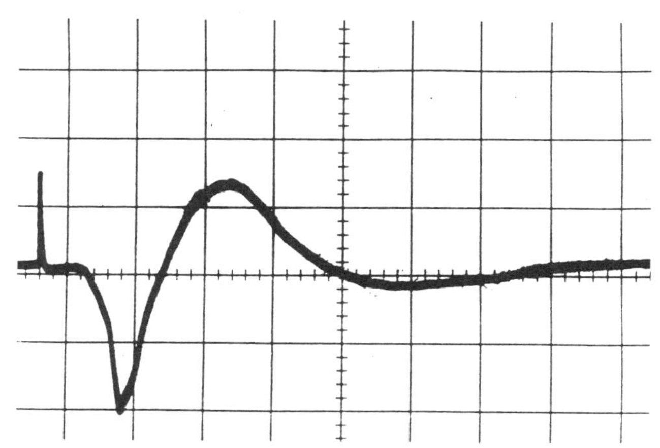

**FIGURE 21.7**
Representative sample of stimulation tracings before interrupting nerve.

In clinical application, Histoacryl® was used in fifty human tympanoplasty procedures: in myringoplasties, ossicular chain, and posterior canal reconstruction. Only minute quantities of the adhesive were used and little inflammation or no reactions were observed. In some cases small amounts were extruded for up to two years after surgery. Only one case—a teenage female diabetic patient—exhibited violent inflammation in the mastoid accompanied by extrusion of Histoacryl®.

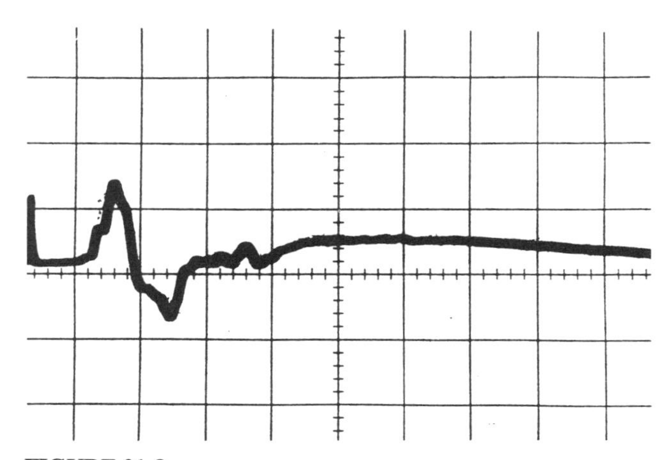

**FIGURE 21.8**
Representative sample of stimulation tracings after nerve repair directly before removal of nerve specimen.

Histoacryl® is still being used in surgical procedures, but since biodegradable fibrin tissue adhesives are available, it would be wiser to discontinue its use entirely.

When it became available, Tisseel®, the commercial pooled donor plasma source fibrin tissue adhesive in experimental surgery, was used on forty-three middle ears of chinchillas. In the first group, one drop of fibrin tissue adhesive was placed on the stapes footplate. In histological sections, the ossicular chain and the middle and inner ear remained undisturbed (Figures 21.9 and 21.10). In the second group, a piece of bone was glued to the long process of the incus. Good bony fusion was observed in all animals. As an example, the organ of Corti, which appears to be well preserved (Figure 21.11), is shown of the animal in Figure 21.10.

From these experiments it was concluded that the commercial fibrin tissue adhesive placed upon the footplate of the stapes is biologically compatible, biodegradable, does not cause toxic, inflammatory or foreign body reactions, or other tissue damage to middle- or inner-ear structures, and that permanent bony fusion was possible.

In another experiment, thirty-four chinchilla ears were tested for tolerance of the inner ear for the commercial fibrin tissue adhesive. The oval window was closed with a connective tissue graft dipped in the adhesive

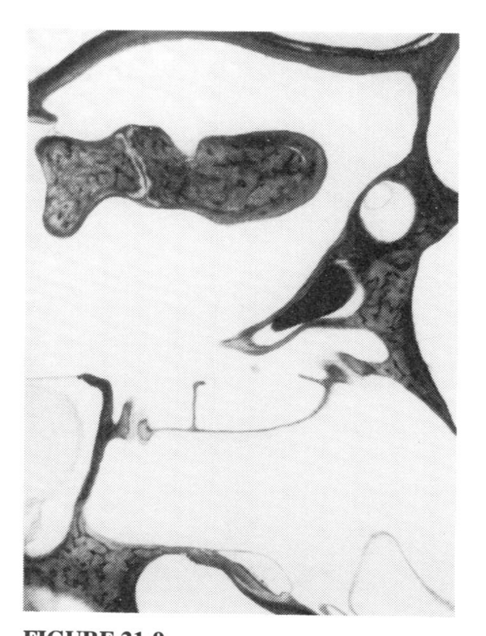

**FIGURE 21.9**
A drop of fibrin adhesive was placed on footplate. Middle-ear and vestibular structures are undisturbed.

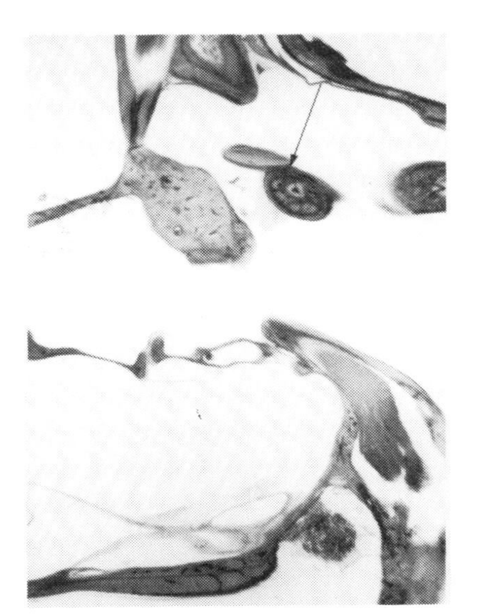

**FIGURE 21.10**
A piece of bone glued to the long process of the incus. Good bony fusion is shown. See arrow.

and a Macor® glass ceramic strut was glued between this graft and the tympanic membrane (Figure 21.12).

The histologic examination did not reveal any inner-ear changes or tissue damage in these animals. The loss in auditory sensitivity monitored by auditory brainstem response thresholds was commensurate with the amount

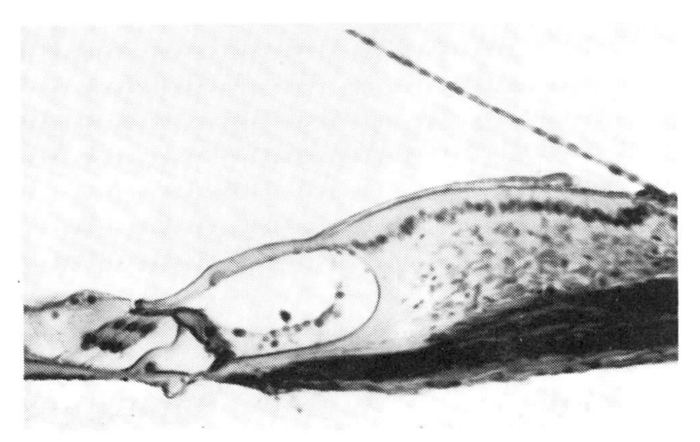

**FIGURE 21.11**
The organ of Corti of animal shown in Figure 21.10 appears well-preserved.

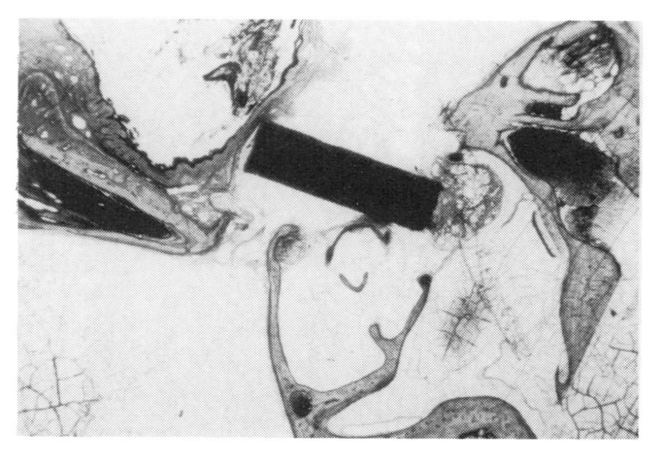

**FIGURE 21.12**
Histologic appearance of middle ear of a chinchilla with the strut healed between fascia graft glued into oval window and tympanic membrane. Stapes had been gently removed. Inner-ear structures are undisturbed.

of loss to be expected with ossicular chain replacement. The findings suggested that this tissue adhesive can be safely applied to the labyrinth (Figures 21.13, 21.14, and 21.15).

Schobel developed a new method of stapedectomy based on the results of research with the Macor® strut implantation in the chinchilla. After partial

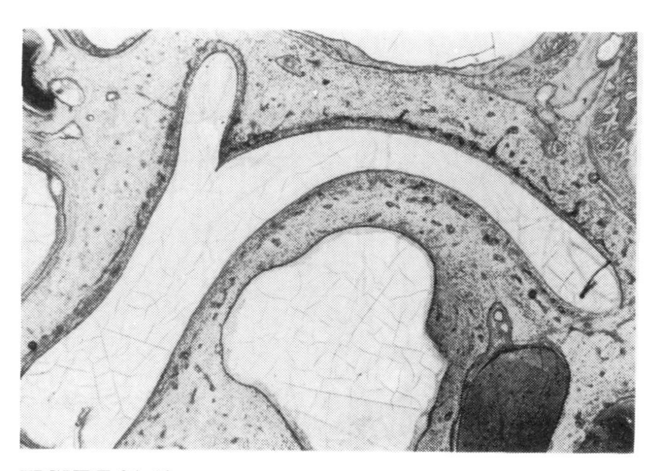

**FIGURE 21.13**
Semicircular canal contents are intact.

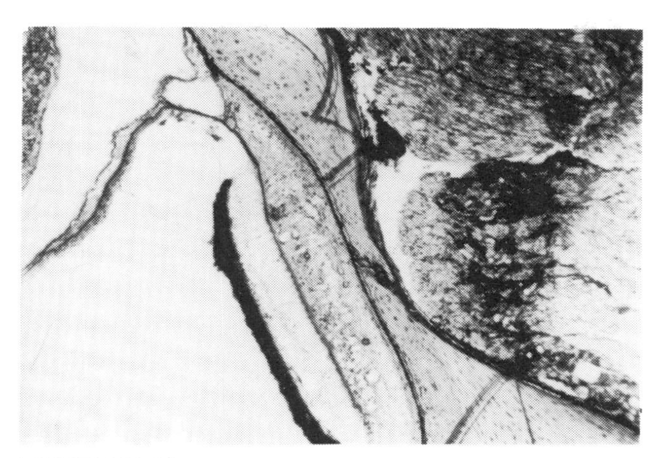

**FIGURE 21.14**
Utricular macula appears normal.

or complete stapes footplate removal, the oval window was glued closed with a fascia graft. A Macor® strut was then glued between the footplate graft and lenticular process (Figure 21.16).

Since the use of fibrin seal is not permitted in the United States because of possible viral transmission, autologous fibrin tissue adhesive (AFTA) was developed. The bonding power of AFTA is directly related to its

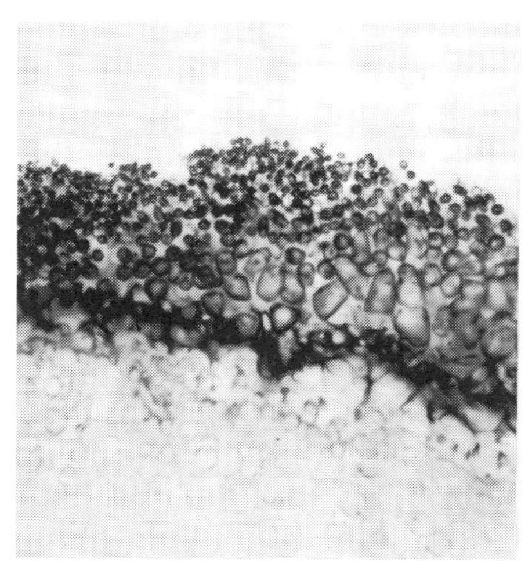

**FIGURE 21.15**
Magnification of utricular macula, showing normal otoconia.

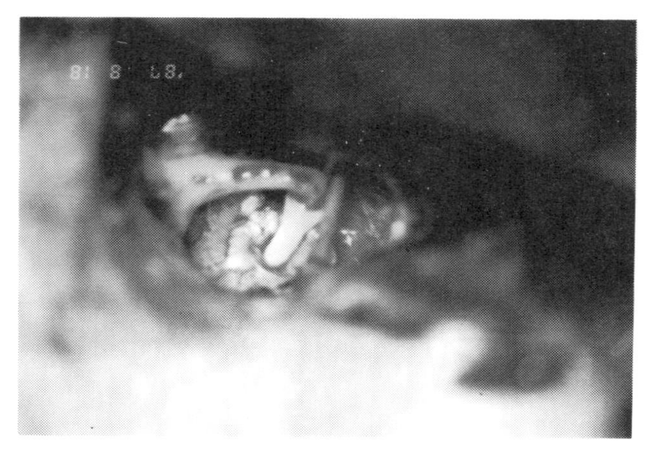

**FIGURE 21.16**
Ceramic strut prosthesis and fascia graft glued into place in human middle ear.

fibrinogen concentration. AFTA was weaker than fibrin sealant ten minutes after bonding, but greater at thirty minutes. Gluing a total ossicular replacement prosthesis (TORP) (Richards) to a 1 $cm^2$ piece of human dura demonstrated greater bonding power when using fibrin sealant (Figures 21.17 and 21.18). Results are summarized in Table 21.1.

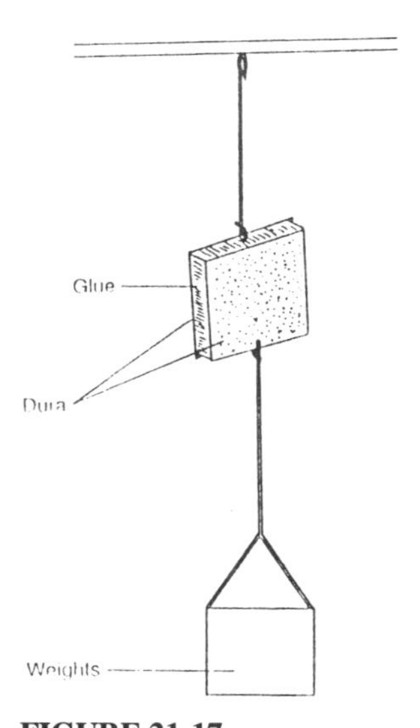


**FIGURE 21.17**
Two 1 $cm^2$ pieces of dura glued with AFTA, suspended and weighted to determine shearing strength of separation.

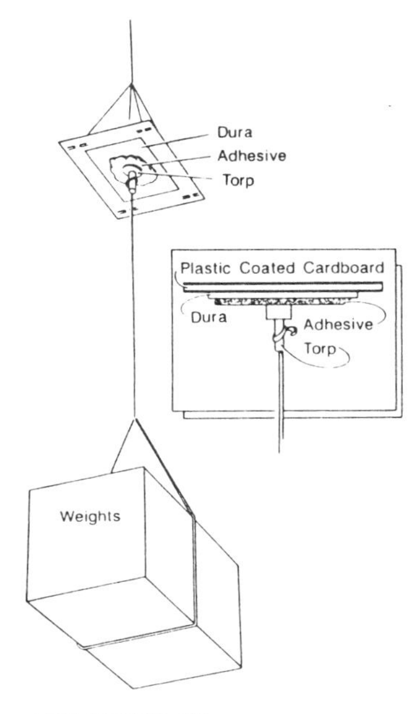


**FIGURE 21.18**
TORP (Richards) glued to 1 $cm^2$ pieces of dura with AFTA, suspended and weighted to determine bonding power at separation.

Autologous fibrin tissue adhesive is combined from two components: one containing fibrinogen and $CaCl_2$ solution and the other containing thrombin solution and epsilon amino caproic acid (EACA) as a fibrinolysis inhibitor. The influence of the inhibitor on the clot dissolution was examined in vitro. The AFTA containing 0, 10, 20 or 30 mg/mL EACA was used. Clots were placed in small specimen jars containing 10 mL Tis-U-Sol® and examined at 1, 3, 7, 14 and 21 days. The jars remained stationary throughout the

***Table 21.1.*** *Bonding strengths of AFTA and FS.*

| | Bond Strength (g) | |
|---|---|---|
| | **AFTA** | **FS** |
| Shearing strength | | |
| Set time: 10 min | 82.5 | 201 |
| 30 min | 380 | 287 |
| TORP bonding strength | | |
| Set time: 10 min | 3.9 | 20.6 |
| 30 min | 7.2 | 43.3 |

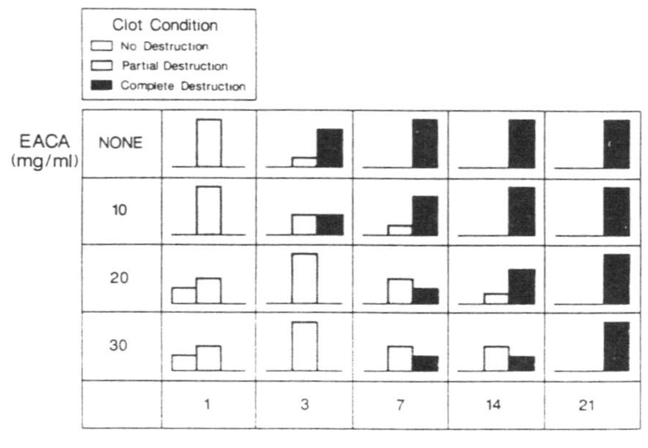


**FIGURE 21.19**
The fibrin adhesive containing no EACA was partially dissolved at three days and completely dissolved at seven days. Partial dissolution occurred at three and seven days in the 10 mg/mL EACA group, and complete dissolution occurred by day fourteen. The 20 mg/mL and 30 mg/mL groups underwent progressive dissolution from three to fourteen days with small fragments of the original clot remaining in both conditions at fourteen days. No clots were found to persist after the twenty-first day.

experiment. Jars containing 0 mg/mL of EACA showed complete dissolution in fourteen days. Jars containing 20 mg/mL of EACA showed complete dissolution in fourteen and twenty-one days and those containing 30 mg/mL of EACA showed complete dissolution in fourteen to twenty-one days. This clearly indicated that the higher the concentration of EACA, the longer the glue clot survived (Figure 21.19).

In vivo fibrinolysis in soft tissue and cartilage was examined by injecting AFTA into rat auricles. Clot survival when using 10 mg/mL of EACA was found to be an average of seven days, while when using 30 mg of EACA it was fourteen days (Figures 21.20 and 21.21). In vivo fibrinolysis examined by injection of AFTA into middle ears of rats revealed that when using 10 mg/mL of EACA four days after injection, middle- and inner-ear structures were not disturbed, and the glue clot was still undissolved in the middle ear (Figure 21.22).

Next, an examination for possible thrombosis due to the use of EACA was made by injecting it intravenously into twenty-four rats, while twelve other rats received only sterile water injections. Autopsy results in all rats receiving intravenous injections of EACA showed no evidence of thrombosis or emboli in major vessels or organ systems. However, areas of hemorrhage were found in all lungs.

The same observations were made on the animals that received equal-

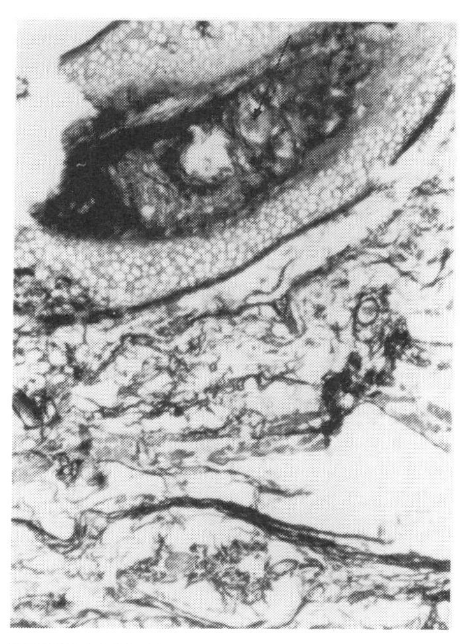

**FIGURE 21.20**
Rat auricle seven days after injection with 0.6 mL of AFTA containing 10 mg EACA. Arrow indicates adhesive clot.

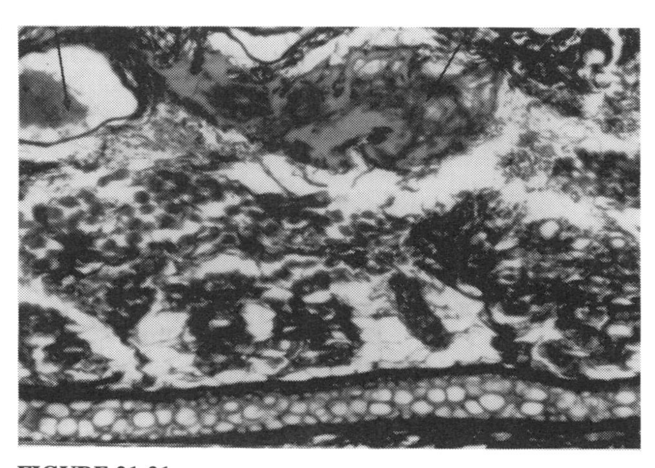

**FIGURE 21.21**
Rat auricle fourteen days after injection with 0.3 mL of AFTA containing 10 mg of EACA. Arrow indicates adhesive clot. No changes in middle ear or labyrinth seen.

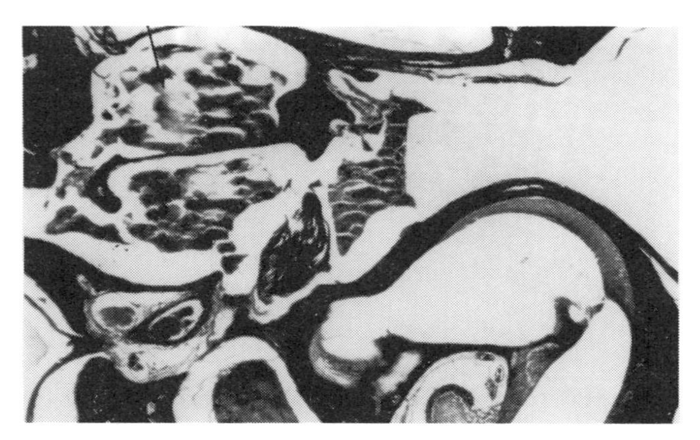

**FIGURE 21.22**
Middle ear of rat four days after injection with 0.3 mL of AFTA containing 10 mg of EACA. Arrow indicates adhesive clot. No changes in middle ear or labyrinth seen.

volume injections of sterile water. Examination of hematoxylin-eosin-stained sections of lungs by a pathologist confirmed the gross pathological findings. Again, control animals showed hemorrhaging only in the lungs. The greatest amount of hemorrhaging was in the group receiving the highest fluid-volume injections. Lung hemorrhaging was deemed to be due to large, intravenous fluid application and not to the fibrinolysis inhibitor.

The AFTA was used in more than 200 cases of middle-ear surgery. It was used for myringoplasties, all types of ossicular chain reconstruction, posterior canal-wall reconstruction, obliteration of attic and mastoid cavities, closure of cerebrospinal fluid leaks with fascia or cartilage, closure of horizontal semicircular canal fistula, and for achievement of hemostasis in cases of severe capillary bleeding.

Others have successfully applied AFTA to close cerebrospinal fluid leaks and to seal fascia grafts for defect repairs in transtemporal acoustic tumor surgery. In facial plastic procedures, skin grafts were securely anchored to the underlying tissues, thus avoiding tissue necrosis. In head and neck cancer surgery, AFTA was used for tissue repair, hemostasis, sealing of incisions, and preventing of seroma formation. Also, frontal sinus cavities have been successfully obliterated with cartilage and fat.

## SUMMARY

This was a description of laboratory, animal, and human surgical experiences with three surgical adhesives, namely Histoacryl® (2-butyl-cyano-acrylate), fibrin seal (fibrin tissue adhesive, Tisseel®), and autologous fibrin tissue adhesive (made from a patient's own blood). Histoacryl® often causes tissue damage and may be subject to extrusion as late as two years after application. Fibrin seal, while entirely biodegradable, is not approved by the Food and Drug Administration because of possible transmission of hepatitis and HIV virus. Autologous fibrin tissue adhesive at present seems to be the best choice for a surgical adhesive in the United States.

## REFERENCES

1. Siedentop, K. H. Reconstruction of ossicles by tissue glue (Histoacryl®) in dogs. *Laryngoscope,* 84:1397–1403, 1974.
2. Siedentop, K. H. Tissue adhesive Histoacryl® (2-butyl-cyano-acrylate) in experimental middle-ear surgery. *Am. J. Otology,* 2:77–87, 1980.
3. Siedentop, K. H., Loewy, A. Facial nerve repair with tissue adhesive. *Arch. Otolaryngology,* 105:423–426, 1979.
4. Siedentop, K. H., Harris, D. M., Loewy, A. Experimental use of fibrin tissue adhesive in middle-ear surgery. *Laryngoscope,* 93: 1310–1313, 1983.
5. Siedentop, K. H., Schobel, H. Stapedectomy modified by the application of fibrin tissue adhesive. *Am. J. Otology,* 12:443–445, 1991.
6. Siedentop, K. H., Harris, D. M., Sanchez, B. Autologous fibrin tissue adhesive: Factors influencing bonding power. *Laryngoscope,* 98:731–733, 1988.
7. Harris, D. M., Siedentop, K. H., Ham, K. R., Sanchez, B. Autologous fibrin tissue adhesive biodegradation and systemic effects. *Laryngoscope,* 97:1141–1144, 1987.

# *Chapter 22: A Review of Nonsuture Peripheral Nerve Repair*

J. K. TERZIS

## INTRODUCTION

When nerve injury occurs, there are many factors involved that collectively determine the clinical outcome. These factors include the age of the patient, how the nerve injury occurred, the extent of damage to the nerve and the surrounding structures, and the time elapsed since the injury. In addition, the immediate environment of the nerve itself plays a role. This includes neurotrophic factors that are produced by the denervated target nerve outflow of axoplasm at the site of injury, ionic shifts in concentrations of extracellular and intracellular fluid (movement of free calcium into axoplasm), and loss of nitrogenous substances from severed fibers into the surrounding media [1].

The evolution of microsurgery has enabled the surgeon to perform microcoaptations of nerves with technical expertise that was impossible even a few decades ago. Although sutures have improved greatly, they are nonbiologic materials that induce an inflammatory response at the repair site. Minimizing scar tissue at the suture line is important in obtaining good healing as well as function [2]. After placement of epineural or perineural stitches, the internal fascicular structure at the suture line becomes disorganized. Misdirection of the regenerating axons is considered one of the most common factors hampering complete nerve function recovery [3]. Therefore, the search continues for alternative methods of nerve repair.

## FIBRIN GLUE

### Historical Review

1940 – Young and Medawar utilized concentrated, coagulated blood plasma fortified with fibrinogen from cockerels for repair of nerve ends [4]. They felt that fiber alignment and growth across the repair site was superior to sutures.

1942 – Seddon and Medawar reported the success of this technique in human nerves [5].

1943 – Tarlov and Benjamin used autologous plasma in rabbits and dogs that caused less inflammation and subsequent fibrosis than cockerels' plasma [6]. They felt that plasma clot sutures were superior to silk sutures, permitting a more precise matching of nerve ends. They showed that the clot was entirely reabsorbed within a few weeks, and that plasma penetration between oppositional surfaces was not deleterious for regeneration. They also showed that when tension existed at the repair site, there was frequent separation of the nerve ends.

1943 – Klemme et al. reported on utilizing cadaver grafts to bridge small gaps [7]. They utilized acacia glue fortified with vitamin B, and an allantoid membrane was placed around the nerve ends.

1944 – Tarlov reported on fourteen patients treated clinically [8]. They reported good results in patients who were followed for an adequate time period.

1945 – Singer used a thin membrane of fibrin from fractionated human plasma with thrombin and fibrinogen and applied this to the cut ends of the nerve [9]. He produced a layer of fibrin around the repair site, creating a tubular sheath. He studied tensile strength as well as tissue response and felt there was increased union strength of union over suture repair.

1972 – Matras et al. used a highly concentrated fibrinogen cryoprecipitate in nerve repair [10]. The glue was placed around the suture line to form a thin cuff with high tensile strength.

Mid 1970s – Duspiva [11], Kuderna [12,13], and Ventura et al. [14] repeated experiments using fibrin clot methods. Kuderna reported that the fibrin clot was equivalent to microsuture techniques.

Late 1970s – Tissucol® or Tisseel® (marketed by Immuno AG, Vienna, Austria) was introduced as a two-component fibrin sealant.

1980s – Egloff and Narakas utilized this two-component system in brachial plexus and nerve trunk repair [15,16]. They published their reports in 1986 on forty-nine of fifty-six patients who had positive results.

1986 – Palazzi presented his experience with fifty-three patients [17].

## Composition of Fibrin Glues

(1) Two-component system (Tissucol® or Tisseel®), consists of 4 IU mL thrombin, human fibrinogen and bovine aprotinin (antifibrinolytic) plus calcium chloride

(2) Tisseel® Duo (500 IU mL thrombin) (otherwise as above)
(3) Autologous fibrinogen utilizes primarily cryoprecipitation techniques to obtain fibrinogen. This eliminates the potential for transmitting hepatitis B and HIV and is mixed with commercially available thrombin preparation and calcium chloride [18]. Another advantage of autologous fibrinogen concentrate is that it does not appear to interfere with the healing process. An increase in fibrinogen concentration correlates with an increase in shear adhesive strength [14].

## Experimental Studies

Several studies looking at various aspects of suture versus fibrin adhesives in nerve repair have been reported. Becker et al. utilized a rat sciatic nerve model to evaluate traumatic degeneration and regeneration in the proximal nerve segment, Wallerian degeneration and regeneration in the distal segment, and atrophy and regeneration of the gastrocnemius and soleus muscles [19]. In all of these parameters no difference between methods was noted. Fibrin did not decrease the traumatic reaction in the proximal nerve stump or improve the recovery of reinnervated muscles.

Cruz et al. [18] divided forty Sprague-Dawley male rats into four groups:

(1) Epineural repairs with six 10-0 interrupted sutures
(2) Epineural repairs with two 10-0 interrupted sutures
(3) Epineural repairs with two 10-0 interrupted sutures reinforced with fibrin glue
(4) Epineural repairs with fibrin glue alone

They found that the addition of fibrin glue to sutures induced greater scar formation and inflammation with distal axonal disorganization. When fibrin glue was used alone, eight showed disruption at eight weeks and two had partial disruption and severe disorganization or regeneration axons. They concluded that fibrin adhesives offer no benefit to conventional suturing and, in addition, is associated with a high dehiscence rate. Other studies have also shown a higher cellular response rate as well as a high dehiscence rate.

Moy et al. looked experimentally at the results of nonabsorbable microsuture versus fibrin seal adhesives (Tissucol®) in repair of the tibial nerve in New Zealand white rabbits [20]. The parameters studied were operating time, clinical function (gait, hindfoot push-off), electrodiagnostic, and histopathology. They noted a decrease in mean amplitude with normal conduction velocities in the Tissucol® group (40% mean amplitude) versus suture group (53% mean amplitude). They felt that this might be indicative of a lag in axonal regeneration in the adhesive group. There was also a higher cellular response in the adhesive group, but they noted that it may have been attributed to the heterologous fibrin used in their experiments. They concluded that the only benefit was a shorter operating time (ten minutes versus seventeen minutes).

Maragh et al. compared microsuture versus fibrin (Tisseel®) in a direct, double-blind study in twenty-five Sprague-Dawley male rats [21]. Tensile strength, electrophysiologic recordings, and morphometric analysis were evaluated. Tensile strength findings at two, four, and eight weeks after surgery demonstrated there was no significant difference between the two repair techniques, although there was a trend toward a stronger hold in the suture group. Electrophysiologic recordings revealed that conventional suture repairs had significantly faster conduction velocities, larger area under the curve, and higher peak amplitudes. The CAP suggest a lower probability of neural regeneration in tissue glue repairs. Although axonal counts proximal and distal to the repair showed no significant difference, there was a suggestion of a higher population of comparable diameter regenerating axons in the suture groups.

Povlsen et al. utilized electron microscopy and noted no statistical difference in nerve regeneration between microsuture repair and the use of Tisseel Duo® in the primary repair of transacted peripheral nerves [22].

Boeckx et al. performed a physiological evaluation of the contraction properties of the innervated gastrocnemius muscle in suture versus fibrin adhesive [23]. Their results indicated a similarity in functional nerve recovery in both groups.

Nishihara and McCaffrey studied (experimentally) fibrin adhesive in nerve grafts as well as neurotomies versus suture [24]. In their study two out of ten nerve grafts repaired with fibrin glue were nonviable and had resorbed, suggesting mechanical dehiscence at the repair site before the establishment of regeneration. In addition, nerve grafts repaired with fibrin adhesive had a significantly lower regenerative index compared to sutured nerves.

Palazzi et al. placed a fibrin sealant block of four millimeters between two ends of the tibialis nerve in the rabbit to study whether this acted as a barrier to block the passage of axons [17]. It was concluded that fibrin adhesive did not act as a barrier to passage of axons across the repair site.

Medders et al. attempted to test the effect of fibrin glue on nerve regeneration by deleting the effects of distraction and/or movement at the anastomosis [25]. Nerve repairs were performed on the intratemporal facial nerve experimentally on albino rats with either fibrin glue or direct approximation without sutures. Fibrin glue was also allowed to become interposed between the nerve ends to determine if the fibrin clot produced a mechanical block to axon regeneration. No significant difference in regenerating axons studied postoperatively (average of forty days) were noted between the two groups, and it was felt that fibrin glue did not produce a mechanical blockage. However, it should be noted that they did not examine the anastomotic site, and could not, therefore, comment histologically on the repair itself.

### Clinical Studies

Sterkers et al. used fibrin glue in repair of the facial nerve in seventy cases and reported Grade III facial regeneration in 62 percent of the cases followed for at least one year [26].

Kanzaki et al. reported satisfactory facial function in two of three patients where the facial nerve had been damaged and repaired by fibrin glue [27].

Narakas utilized fibrin glue in repair of peripheral nerves by creating a cylinder of glue four times as long as the diameter of the nerve [28,29]. In addition, one or two sutures were used. The glue was used clinically since 1980 in repair of motor nerves, such as axillary, suprascapular, and musculocutaneous. They reported no failures and observed 25 percent more cases with results better than with sutures alone. They felt that fibrin sealant shortened operative time, allowed an easier stabilization of the apposition obtained, and possibly improved the result.

Although reported experimentally and clinically to decrease operating time, little conclusive evidence has been shown of benefit of fibrin glue over conventional microsuture repair. Many studies have noted a high dehiscence rate when fibrin sealant is used. Although perhaps providing a barrier to axonal sprouting, this may be counterbalanced by a possible increase in the inflammatory response. Autologous fibrin may provide a means of increasing shear adhesive strength and decreasing the fibroblastic response. Further experimental and clinical studies need to be done to evaluate the immunologic responses to fibrin glues. Studies directed toward improving the tensile strength of autologous fibrinogen components should be performed as well.

## CYANOACRYLATES

Cyanoacrylates were first synthesized in 1949 by Ardis [30]. It is possible to alter the cyanoacrylate compound by altering the alkoxycarbornyl group (−COOR). Coover suggested the usage of cyanoacrylates as surgical adhesives [31]. Methyl-2-cyanoacrylate (Eastman 910 monomer) was the first derivative marketed as a surgical adhesive. Longer chain derivatives, such as ethyl-2-cyanoacrylate (Krazy Glue®), isobutyl-2-cyanoacrylate (Bucrylate®), and butyl-2-cyanoacrylate (Histoacryl®) have subsequently been developed. The shorter chain derivatives (methyl- and ethyl-) have shown to have greater histotoxicity than the longer chain derivatives (isobutyl- and butyl-).

Early studies have shown the unsuitability of the short chain derivatives in attempting peripheral nerve repair. Ferlic and Goldner utilized methyl 2-cyanoacrylate to anastomose the cut ends of twenty-two posterior tibial nerves in rabbits [32]. Only seven showed any evidence of union and also demonstrated unsatisfactory axonal regeneration. All of the nerve repairs showed degeneration and necrosis. Nerve damage was caused by the heat given off at the time the material polymerizes.

Braun showed experimentally that alkyl 2-cyanoacrylate was associated with an adverse tissue response histologically [33]. This included both large and small mononuclear cells. In addition, the inclusion of adhesive between the cut ends prevented successful nerve repair.

Wlodarczyk injected Histoacryl® into a gap of the isolated frog nerve and noted the abolishment of the compound action potential [34].

In contrast to the above reports, Mielke reported favorably on the use of Histoacryl® for clinically grafting the interrupted recurrent nerve [35].

Siedentop and Loewy looked at facial nerves in dogs, which were repaired by either epineural sutures with a silastic sheath wrapped around the repair site or a tissue adhesive (Histoacryl® ) [36]. Successful repair was defined as (1) the observation of motion in the muscles that were innervated after electrical stimulation of the nerve proximal to the repair site, and (2) evaluation of microanatomical continuity by histopathological means. The results were equivalent in both groups and both electroconductivity and microanatomic continuity were present. They concluded that adhesive was easier to use and less time consuming.

It should also be noted that the degradation of cyanoacrylate derivatives yield the tissue toxic by-products cyanoacetate and formaldehyde [37,38]. Shorter chain derivatives degrade faster and therefore release their by-products to produce a higher tissue concentration. The by-products of the longer chain derivatives can be more readily cleared by the host tissues. The development of sarcomas in rats after subcutaneous injections of large doses of methyl-2-cyanoacrylate has been reported [39]. Methyl-2-cyanoacrylate was subsequently banned for clinical use by the Food and Drug Administration. Other studies have failed to show carcinogenesis with butyl- and isobutyl-derivatives [40,41]. Histoacryl®, however, is not available in the United States.

## LASER WELDING OF NERVES

Another alternative to microsuture repair of peripheral nerves is laser repair. One theoretical advantage is that laser does not introduce foreign material into the anastomotic site. Various techniques have been described regarding welding of nerve tissue. This includes circumferential welding, creating a sheath with either epineural or local subcutaneous tissue, or utilizing red blood cells as a vector. Four different types of lasers have been used in nerve repair. These are the $CO_2$, KTP, argon and YAG lasers. The YAG laser has been shown to cause endoneural damage and is generally not used [42]. It is believed that the mechanism of tissue welding by laser is through homogenizing epineural collagen. Most perineural cells are preserved. The thermal force produces a denaturation and fusion process in protein molecules.

Fisher et al. attempted neural anastomosis using the $CO_2$ laser [43]. They reported that laser repair produced less scar-tissue formation and constriction at the repair site. However, laser repair requires precise control of the thermal effects to permit welding of the epineurium without damage to the underlying axons.

### Experimental Studies

Maragh et al. compared $CO_2$ laser nerve repair to microsuture coaptation experimentally in thirty-five Sprague-Dawley male rats [44]. They evaluated tensile strength and functional assessment utilizing electrophysiologic recordings, toe spread, and quantitative morphology. They did not utilize any ancillary techniques to aid in the repair. The results showed no dehiscence in the suture group versus a 12% dehiscence rate in the laser group. In addition, the amount of laser energy at the repair site reduced the rate of dehiscence.

The tensile-strength findings confirmed that at four days microsuture repair was significantly stronger, but thereafter, there was no difference between the two techniques. Histologically, both techniques allowed axons to cross the repair site. Distally, no differences were noted between the two groups; however, proximally there were more fine, myelinated fibers in the suture group as well as a foreign body response. Electrophysiologic studies showed significantly faster conduction velocities for the suture group, but the area of the wave forms of the peak amplitudes showed no statistical significant differences.

Huang et al. also compared (experimentally) laser versus suture nerve anastomosis utilizing $CO_2$ circumferential welding plus the addition of two anchoring sutures [45]. They found that although laser repair took less time, there was a high rate of dehiscence (41%) in the laser group, while there was no dehiscence in the suture group. Anatomically they noted no adverse effects on axonal regeneration, either antegrade or retrograde, and no evidence of deep thermal penetration or external scarring. There were no statistical differences of functional recovery between the two groups.

Kim and Kline used a strip of peri-epineural sheath wrapped around distal and proximal stumps to supplement $CO_2$ laser welding and compared the results to microsuture repair [46]. They reported no dehiscences in either group. The suture group had more evidence of scarring while the laser group showed very little proliferation of connective tissue. Both groups showed ingrowth of blood vessels and good distal regeneration. There were no statistically significant differences electrophysiologically between the two groups. They concluded that peri-epineural laser repair decreases tension at the anastomotic site and increases tensile strength. They also felt that this technique avoided intraneural damage because the welding occurs proximal and distal to the transection site. There was less axonal escape noted in the peri-epineural repair group.

Korff et al. compared a two-suture epineural repair with a subcutaneous tissue weld (S-Q weld) technique [42]. They showed nine of fifteen repairs with dehiscence in the laser group versus one of fifteen in the suture group. They felt that the S-Q weld technique showed greater tensile strength than welding at the anastomosis alone, but less than the suture group. Although not statistically significant, electrophysiologic and histologic evaluation of regeneration in repaired nerves showed a greater number of regenerating axons in the laser group. Histologically there were no significant differences between the number of axons or population in the two groups.

Finally, Almquist evaluated the use of argon laser in repairing rat and primate nerves [47]. Utilizing rat sciatic nerves, blood was placed around the anastomotic site and coagulated with the argon laser. During coagulation, they noted that some heat was transferred to adjacent axonal tissue, but there were no apparent changes within perineural structures. Scanning electron microscropy showed early axonal budding at the repair site that proceeded distally. However, there was no attempt to quantify nerve regeneration. No undue fibrosis was noted at the repair site.

The seal formed by laser repair is circumferential and helps prevent fibroblasts from invading the repair site or axon sprouts to escape. The technique also avoids trauma introduced by needles and has the advantage of not utilizing foreign needles to achieve coaptation. Laser welding also may prove to take significantly less time than microsuture repair.

However, due to the problems of decreased tensile strength and increased dehiscence rates, welding has not been found to be superior to microsuture repair, although utilizing techniques that create a sheath around the repair site may aid in decreasing tension and therefore decrease the dehiscence rate. Further investigations are needed to study the effects of lasers on nerve repair as well as the long term effectiveness of laser over microsuture repair.

## CELL SURGERY IN NERVE REPAIR

In 1983 de Medinacelli introduced a technique of nerve repair, termed "reconnection," that was shown to yield satisfactory functional results in animals [48]. The principles of this "cell surgery" involve precise repair at the cellular level by attempting to minimize the chemical damage that occurs with nerve disruption. This minimizes the physical damage that occurs with attempts at nerve repair and obtaining a tension-free microcoaptation.

More recently a preliminary report on ten clinical cases has been reported [49]. The general surgical technique involves adding a chlorpromazine hydrochloride solution to the nerve stumps before dissection to help protect the nerve against the adverse effects of free calcium ions. A modified Collins solution is added as well prior to controlled freezing of the stumps to minimize the stress of freezing. Prior to freezing, the stumps are sutured to a support of bioabsorbable material with overlapping of the nerve ends. After freezing, the stumps are trimmed with a sharp blade. In three of ten cases, fibrin glue was added to the repair site to secure the anastomosis since the use of a tourniquet prevented fibrin clot formation. No other sutures were utilized. The preliminary reports in nine of ten cases were encouraging, even in cases in which there were poor local conditions with associated vascular lesions, or poor health of the patient.

Terzis and Smith experimentally compared the de Medinacelli method with standard microsurgical methods [50]. It was shown that the return of function was significantly better in nerves severed and repaired with the reconnection technique than when severed and repaired with conventional microsuture techniques. The improvement was attributed to a more accurate realignment of the severed stumps in the reconnection technique, rather than to an improvement in the numbers or rate of growth of the regenerated fibers, which was similar in both groups.

However, at the present time, the "cell-surgery" technique is complex and cannot be used without proper and reliable equipment. In addition, the technique is difficult to apply clinically [49]. Currently, technical improvements are being worked on that may lead to further clinical studies.

## THE FUTURE

Current microsurgical techniques afford precise repair of nerves at the fascicular level. The next step is to gain precision at the axonal as well as the cellular level. Advancement through a greater understanding of neurochemistry and neurobiology will be the next logical step in nerve repair.

## REFERENCES


1. de Medinacelli, L., Freed, W. J., Wyatt, R. J. Peripheral nerve reconnection: Improvement of long-term functional effects under simulated clinical conditions in the rat. *Exp. Neurol.*, 81:488–496, 1983.
2. Bently, F. H., Hill, M. Experimental surgery: Nerve grafting. *Br. J. Surg.*, 24:368–372, 1936.
3. Bertelli, J. A., Mira, J. C. Nerve repair using freezing and fibrin glue: Immediate histologic improvement of axonal coaptation. *Mircosurg.*, 14:135–140, 1993.
4. Young, J. Z., Medawar, P. B. Fibrin suture of peripheral nerves: Measurement of the rate of regeneration. *The Lancet,* 2:126, 1940.
5. Seddon, H. J., Medawar, P. B. Fibrin suture of human nerves. *The Lancet,* 2:87–88, 1942.
6. Tarlov, I. M., Benjamin, B. Plasma clot and silk suture of nerves: An experimental study of comparative tissue reaction. *Surg. Gynecol. Obstet.,* 76:366, 1943.
7. Klemme, R. M., Woolsoy, R. D., DeRezend, N. T. Autopsy nerve grafts in peripheral nerve surgery. *JAMA,* 122:393, 1943.
8. Tarlov, I. M. Autologous plasma clot suture of nerves: Its use in clinical surgery. *JAMA,* 126:741, 1944.
9. Singer, M. The combined use of fibrin film and clot in end-to-end union nerves: An experimental study. *J. Neurosurg.*, 2:102, 1945.
10. Matras, H., Dinges, H. P., Manoli, B., et al. Nonsutured nerve transplantation. *J. Maxillofac. Surg.*, 1:37–40, 1973.
11. Duspiva, W. Neue erkenntnisse zur anastomosierung durchtrennter peripherer nerven. *Forster. Med.*, 93, 43:2214–2218, 1975.
12. Kuderna, H. Nervenklebung. *Dtsche. Zahn-Mund-Kiefer-Gesichtschri.*, 3:32, 1979.
13. Kuderna, H. Klinische anwendung der klebung von nerven: Anastomsoen mit fibrinogen. *Fortschritte d. Kiefer u. Gesichtschri.*, 21:135, 1976.
14. Ventura, G., Torri, G., Campari, A., et al. Experimental suture of the peripheral nerves with "fibrin-glue." *Ital. J. Orthop. Traumatol.*, 6:407, 1980.
15. Egloff, D. V., Narakas, A. Nerve anastomosis with human fibrin: Preliminary clinical report (56 cases). *Ann. Chir. Main.*, 21:101, 1983.
16. Egloff, D. V., Narakas, A., Bonnard, C. Results of nerve grafts with Tissucol® (Tisseel®) anastomosis. In: *Fibrin Sealant in Operative Medicine. Ophthalmology Neurosurgery,* Vol. 2, G. Schlag and H. Redl, eds. Berlin: Springer-Verlag, 1986.
17. Palazzi, S., Vila-Torres, J. Lorenzo, J. C. Fibrin glue is a sealant and not a nerve barrier. Update and future trends in fibrin sealing in surgical and nonsurgical fields. Presented at Hotel Hilton, AM Stadtpart, Nov. 15–18, 1992.
18. Cruz, N. I., Bebs, N., Fiol, R. E. Evaluation of fibrin glue in rat sciatic nerve repairs. *Plast. Reconstr. Surg.*, 73(3):369–373, 1986.

19. Becker, C. M., Gueuning, C. O., Graff, G. L. Status of fibrin glue for divided rat nerves: Schwaan cell and muscle metabolism. *Microsurgery,* 6:1 – 10, 1985.
20. Moy, O. J., Peimer, C. A., Koniuch, M. P., et al. Fibrin seal adhesive versus nonabsorbable microsuture in peripheral nerve repair. *J. Hand Surg.,* 13A:273 – 278, 1988.
21. Maragh, H. Meyer, B. S., Davenport, D., Gould, J. D., Terzis, J. K. Morphofunctional evaluation of fibrin glue versus microsuture nerve repairs. *J. Reconstr. Microsurg.,* 6(4):331 – 337, 1990.
22. Povlsen, B., Danielsson, P., Nylander, G. Fibrin in the primary repair of transsected peripheral nerves. Update and future trends in fibrin sealing in surgical and nonsurgical fields. Presented at Hotel Hilton, AM Stadtpart Nov. 15 – 18, 1992.
23. Boeckx, W., Stockmans, F., Guelinckx, P. Microsurgical and physiological evaluation of nerve repair with microsuture versus tissue adhesive. Update and future trends in fibrin sealing in surgical and nonsurgical fields. Presented at Hotel Hilton, AM Stadtpart Nov. 15 – 18, 1992.
24. Nishihira, S., McCaffrey, T. V. Repair of motor nerve defects: Comparison of suture and fibrin adhesive techniques. *Otolaryngol. Head Neck Surg.,* 100:17, 1989.
25. Medders, G., Mattox, D. E., Lyles A. Effects of fibrin glue on rat facial nerve regeneration. *Otolaryngol. Head Neck Surg.,* 100:106, 1989.
26. Sterkers, O., Julien, N., Sterkers, J. M. Fibrin glue anastomosis of the facial nerve. Update and future trends in fibrin sealing in surgical and nonsurgical fields. Presented at Hotel Hilton, AM Stadtpart Nov. 15 – 18, 1992.
27. Kanzaki, J., Kunihiro, T., Ouchi, T., et al. Intracranial reconstruction of the facial nerve. *Acta Otolaryngol. Suppl.,* 487:85 – 90, 1991.
28. Narakas, A. The use of fibrin glue in repair of peripheral nerves. *Ortho. Clinics North Am.,* 19:187 – 199, 1988.
29. Narakas, A. O., Bonnard, C. H. Ten years experience using Tissucol® for the repair of brachial plexus. Update and future trends in fibrin sealing surgical and nonsurgical fields. Presented at Hotel Hilton, AM Stadtpart Nov. 15 – 18, 1992.
30. Ardis, A. E., U.S. Patents 2467926 and 2467927 (1949).
31. Coover, H. W., Joyner, F. B., Shearer, N. H., et al. Chemistry and performance of cyanoacrylate adhesives. *J. Soc. Plast Eng.,* 15:413 – 417, 1959.
32. Ferlic, D. C., Goldner, J. L. Evaluation of the effect of methyl-2-cyanoacrylate (Eastman 910 Monomer) on peripheral nerves. *South. Med. Journ.,* 58:679 – 685, 1965.
33. Braun, R. M. Comparative studies of neurorrhaphy and sutureless peripheral nerve repair. *Surgery Gynec. Obstet.,* 122:15 – 18, 1966.
34. Wlodarczyk, J. Effects of tissue glues on electrical activity in isolated nerve. *Polim. Med.,* 21:37 – 41, 1991.
35. Mielke, A. Probleme bei der naht der feinten peripheren nerven in bereich der oto-laryngologie. *Melsunger med. Mitteilung.,* 42:71 – 74, 1968.
36. Siedentop, K. H., Loewy, A. Facial nerve repair with tissue adhesives. *Arch. Otolaryngol.,* 105:423 – 426, 1979.
37. Toriumi, D. M., Raslan, W. F., Friedman, M., et al. Variable histotoxicity of

Histoacryl® when used in a subcutaneous site: An experimental study. *Laryngoscope,* 101:339–343, 1991.

38. Toriumi, D. M., Raslan, W. F., Friedman, M., et al. Histotoxicity of cyanoacrylate tissue adhesives. *Arch. Otolaryngol. Head Neck Surg.*, 116:546–550, 1990.
39. Samson, D., Marshall, D. Carcinogenic potential of isobutyl-2-cyanoacrylate. *J. Neurosurg.*, 65:571–572, 1986.
40. Lehman, RAW, Hayes, G. J., Leonard, F. Toxicity of alkyl 2-cyanoacrylates, I: peripheral nerve. *Arch. Surg.*, 93:441–446, 1966.
41. Matsumoto, T., HisterKamp, C. A. Long-term study of aerosol cyanoacrylate tissue adhesive spray: Carcinogenicity and other untoward effects. *Ann. Surg.*, 25:825–827, 1969.
42. Korff, M., Brent, S. W., Havig, M. T., et al. An investigation of the potential for laser nerve welding. *Otol. Head Neck Surg.*, 106:345–350, 1992.
43. Fischer, D. W., Beggs, J. L., Kenshalo, D. L., et al. Comparative study of microepineural anastomosis with the use of $CO_2$ laser and suture techniques in rat sciatic nerves. Part 1. *Neurosurg.*, 17:300, 1985.
44. Maragh, H., Hawn, R. S., Gould, J. P., Terzis, J. K. Is laser nerve repair comparable to microsuture coaptation? *J. Recons. Microsurg.*, 413:189–195, 1988.
45. Huang, T. C., Blanks, R. H. I, Berns, M. W., et al. Laser versus suture nerve anastomosis. *Otol. Head Neck Surg.*, 107:14–20, 1992.
46. Kim, D. H., Kline, D. G. Peri-epineural tissue to supplement laser welding of nerve. *Neurosurgery,* 26:211–216, 1990
47. Almquist, E., Nachemson, A., Auth, D., et al. Evaluation of the use of the argon laser in repairing rat and primate nerves. *J. Hand Surg.*, 9A:792–799, 1984.
48. de Medinacelli, L., Wyatt, R. J., Freed, W. J. Peripheral nerve reconnection: Mechanical, thermal, and ionic conditions that promote the return of function. *Exp. Neurol.*, 81:469–487, 1983.
49. de Medinacelli, L., Merle, M. Applying "cell surgery" to nerve repair: A preliminary report of the first ten human cases. *J. Hand Surg.*, 16B:499–504, 1991.
50. Terzis, J. K., Smith K. J. Repair of severed peripheral nerves: Comparison of the "de Medinacelli" and standard microsuture methods. *Exp. Neurol.*, 96:672–680, 1987.

# *Chapter 23: Clinical Use of Fibrin-Based Composite Tissue Adhesive in Otology and Neurotology*

**R. C. PERKINS and D. H. SIERRA**

## INTRODUCTION

Fibrin sealant (FS) has been used successfully in a number of head and neck surgical indications, incorporating microsurgical techniques, in particular otology and neurotology. The use of both highly concentrated, pooled-source commercial FS (Tissucol®) [1,2] and patient autologous FS [3,4] has been documented. Patient autologous FS produced by cryoprecipitation quickly demonstrated shortcomings in certain performance characteristics, specifically cohesive and adhesive strength as well as low viscosity prior to polymerization (gelation).

The last characteristic especially impeded the utility of FS in otologic reconstructive procedures such as ossiculoplasties. The adhesive would invariably migrate from the repair site regardless if both components, fibrinogen and thrombin, were applied in sequence or simultaneously. Increasing the thrombin or fibrinogen concentrations had little effect. Strength was a concern when FS was applied in neurotological procedures to obtain fluid continence when the dura mater was transected. These challenges led to the development of a fibrin-collagen composite tissue adhesive (CTA). The in vitro development is described in another chapter [5].

## CLINICAL TRIALS

A pilot, human clinical trial was conducted to evaluate the utility and efficacy of two CTA formulations. The trial was not intended to be a rigorously controlled investigation but to determine where CTA would perform best for a range of procedures. These results would later be used in the development of a controlled clinical study of surgical procedure where the adhesive was found most useful.

Human clinical trials included thirty patients undergoing a variety of otologic and neurotologic procedures. The cases were broken down into two phases. Phase I incorporated the use of patient autologous cryoprecipitate [6] with collagen, thrombin, and $\epsilon$-aminocaproic acid. Twenty-one subjects were assigned to this phase. Phase II incorporated the use of patient autologous plasma (citrated) with collagen, thrombin, and $\epsilon$-aminocaproic acid.

## Patients

Thirty patients, sixteen males and fourteen females, with an average age of forty-one years (range nine to sixty-eight years) were enrolled in the study. They were candidates for a range of otologic and head and neck neurotologic procedures requiring conventional repair and closure techniques. Patient participation in this study was voluntary; informed consent was obtained. Patients with a known hypersensitivity to bovine source products were excluded.

## Investigational Materials

The CTA is comprised of two components: the first consists of fibrous atelopeptide type I bovine collagen compounded with patient autologous fibrinogen and Factor XIII; the second, a bovine thrombin solution reconstituted in dilute $CaCl_2$ and $\epsilon$-aminocaproic acid. Two formulations of the CTA were evaluated (see Table 23.1).

The collagen is mixed with the fibrinogen prior to the start of the procedure (component 1). The mixture is then combined sequentially via

***Table 23.1.*** *Composite tissue adhesive formulations.*

| Formulation | [Fibrinogen] (mg/mL, nominal) | Source |
|---|---|---|
| CTA-I | 15 | cryoprecipitate |
| CTA-II | 1.5 | plasma |
| | **for both formulations:** | |
| | [collagen]: 18 mg/mL<br>[thrombin]: 200 U/mL<br>[$CaCl_2$]: 20 mM<br>[$\epsilon$-aminocaproic acid]: 25 mg/mL<br>amount component 1 made: 1 mL | |

syringes with thrombin-$CaCl_2$-antifibrinolytic (component 2) at the site of repair.

### Neurotologic Procedures

The CTA was used primarily to close and seal the dura and cranial bone subsequent to the removal of acoustic neuromas or the repair of encephaloceles. For acoustic neuroma procedures the internal auditory canal was packed with autogenous fat and muscle coated with CTA after the removal of the tumor. This was followed by placing a layer of CTA over the packing, and in the case of the encephalocele repair, a piece of homograft dura was secured over the closure. In both procedures, the dura was patched with a piece of homograft dura sutured into place, then sealed about the periphery with CTA. The objective was to obtain a cerebrospinal fluid-tight seal during closure.

### Otologic Procedures

The tympanossicular chain reconstruction procedures required microsurgical techniques to repair or replace the various components of the middle ear. The CTA was used to position and hold the replacement components (tympanic membrane, ossicles, prostheses, etc.) in the desired anatomic configuration without the use of absorbable packing. In the mastoid bone/canal reconstructions, CTA was mixed with autogenous bone tissue and in conjunction with homograft dura was used to rebuild the middle-ear and canal wall. This was performed after the removal of infected and damaged bone and soft tissue. The epithelium and tympanic membrane were fixed to the rebuilt canal and mastoid with CTA. In the external ear reconstruction procedures, the meatus was enlarged and recontoured by making a series of incisions about the canal opening to remove portions of native cartilagenous structures. The skin flaps were repositioned and held in place with CTA. The gaps between the flaps were also filled and contoured with the adhesive.

### Evaluation Procedure

Patients were evaluated weekly for four weeks postoperatively, then monthly thereafter. In the first four weeks, the treatment site was assessed for tissue reactions including erythema, swelling, induration and inflammation. For neurological procedures, cerebrospinal fluid continence was evaluated. For otologic procedures, the impact of CTA in the reconstruction and replacement of bony elements as well as improvement in hearing performance was evaluated.

***Table 23.2.*** *Number of neurotologic and otologic procedures per formulation.*

| | Formulation | |
|---|---|---|
| **Procedure** | **CTA-I** | **CTA-II** |
| Acoustic neuroma | 0 | 3 |
| Encephalocele repair | 0 | 1 |
| Tympanossicular chain repair | 19 | 2 |
| Mastoid/canal wall repair | 4 | 0 |
| External ear reconstruction | 1 | 0 |
| Totals: | 24 | 6 |

## Clinical Results

A total of thirty patients were treated with both CTA formulations. A summary of the procedures and formulations used are presented in Table 23.2.

There were no indications of inflammation or delay in healing compared to cases with typical closure and repair techniques. In the case of external ear reconstruction, CTA appeared to promote good re-epithelialization between the skin flaps with no apparent scarring. The patient with tympanossicular chain repair regained hearing at rates and ranges expected for those procedures.

During the neurological procedures, and in subsequent postsurgical evaluation, the adhesive was an effective fluid-tight barrier. It had good adhesive and mechanical strength, firmly holding the tissue in the desired configurations. The CTA was viscous and easily moldable and immediately set-up upon the addition of thrombin solution. This feature facilitated microsurgical reconstructive and replacement techniques. The CTA reduced or obviated the need for external pressure packing, allowing for earlier observation of the post surgical healing process.

There was no obvious difference in clinical performance between the two formulations. The CTA was considered subjectively to perform better than cryoprecipitated FS. No migration from the repair sites was observed in any of the procedures or when packing was secured more firmly in place when pulled. Failures in securing packing were noted in cases utilizing FS.

## CONCLUSIONS

Head and neck surgical procedures require a variety of techniques for the repair and replacement of damaged and missing anatomic features. In many instances, conventional repair and closure techniques are inadequate due to limited accessibility of the repair sites even with current microsurgical techniques.

The pilot evaluation of CTA for neurologic and otologic procedures demonstrated the utility, flexibility, and efficacy of the fibrin-based technology in a number of different clinical indications. The CTA proved to be a useful and a valuable adjunct to microsurgery by acting as a tissue adhesive, fluid-tight sealant, hemostatic agent, and packing material.

Postoperative follow-up for up to seven years for patients treated with CTA indicated that the adhesive is biocompatible and clinically effective in a wide variety of roles. No untoward effects were observed in any of the patients. Clinical assessment of the material indicates that this material is a valuable addition to existing surgical techniques.

## ACKNOWLEDGEMENTS

The authors wish to thank Drs. Alan Nissen and Joseph Welch for their participation in these studies. We also wish to thank the staff at the California Ear Institute at Stanford and Project Hear for their assistance and support. Many thanks to Joseph Roberson, M.D. for reviewing this manuscript.

## REFERENCES

1. Staindl, O. Tissue adhesion with highly concentrated human fibrinogen in otolaryngology. *Ann. Otol. Rhinol. Laryngol.*, 88:413–418, 1979.
2. Schlag, G., Redl, H., eds. Fibrin sealant in operative medicine. Vol 1. *Otorhinolaryngology.* Springer-Verlag, Berlin. 1986.
3. Siedentop, K. H., Harris, D. M., Ham, K., Sanchez, B. Extended experimental and preliminary surgical findings with autologous fibrin tissue adhesive made from patient's own blood. *Laryngoscope,* 96:1062–1064, 1986.
4. Epstein, G. H., Weisman, R. A., Zwillenberg, S., Schreiber, A. D. A new autologous fibrinogen-based adhesive for otologic surgery. *Ann Otol. Rhinol. Laryngol.*, 95:40–45, 1986.
5. Sierra, D. H. Fibrin-collagen composite tissue adhesive. In: *Surgical Adhesives and Sealants: Current Technology and Applications.* D. H. Sierra and R. Saltz, eds. Technomic Publishing Company, Inc., Lancaster, PA, 1996.
6. Sierra, D. H., Nissen, A. J. Welch, J. The use of fibrin glue in intracranial procedures: Preliminary results. *Laryngoscope,* 100:360–363, 1990.

# *Chapter 24: Clinical Applications of Fibrin Sealant in Thoracic and Cardiovascular Surgery*

W. D. SPOTNITZ

## INTRODUCTION

The specialty of thoracic and cardiovascular surgery (TCV) has developed rapidly during the second half of the twentieth century. Use of the cardiopulmonary by-pass has allowed for the surgical treatment of many congenital and acquired forms of cardiovascular disease. Large numbers of patients with atherosclerotic coronary artery disease, in particular, have been treatable with surgical intervention using coronary-artery by-pass grafting. The rapid growth in the cardiopulmonary by-pass procedures, which require anticoagulation with heparin, has increased the need for effective hemostatic agents to reduce the incidence of postoperative hemorrhage.

For this purpose, fibrin sealant is gaining increased popularity as a surgical tissue adhesive. Its widespread use in this country, despite the absence of a commercially available Food and Drug Administration approved-product label is quite remarkable.

Many of the major thoracic and cardiovascular surgical centers in the country have mechanisms for obtaining concentrated sources of human fibrinogen and Factor XIII required with bovine thrombin and calcium for the formation of fibrin tissue adhesive. Sources include single-donor plasma, fresh-frozen plasma, cryoprecipitate, and autologous whole blood. A variety of cryoprecipitation and chemical processes are available to enhance fibrinogen concentrations.

## UNIVERSITY OF VIRGINIA SYSTEM

At the University of Virginia Health Sciences Center in Charlottesville, a single-donor cryoprecipitation process has been used since 1985 [1]. The individual units of fibrinogen are tracked and documented for each donor and recipient. Serologic donor testing includes hepatitis B surface antigen and antibody, hepatitis B core antibody, hepatitis C antibody, and HIV antibody in order to reduce the risk of blood-borne disease transmission. This system has been used in more than 2200 patients over the past eight years. More than 1300 of these patients have undergone TCV operations with no documented episodes of viral disease transmission. The same system is also in place for autologous donation when clinical conditions permit its use.

## METHODS OF APPLICATION

Making fibrin sealant easily and rapidly available to thoracic and cardiovascular surgeons at the University of Virginia Health Sciences Center has fostered a variety of new application methods. The most widely used technique involves the use of spray bottles and is highly effective for assuring adequate mixing of fibrinogen and thrombin over large surface areas [2]. Individual, blunt-nosed cannulas on the end of syringes can also be used for the application of the two-component, fibrin-sealant system to discrete suture lines.

Areas of more rapid active bleeding can be treated using a carrier sponge of collagen or cellulose to deliver the fibrin sealant. The sponge is first soaked in fibrinogen and then activated with thrombin spray just prior to positioning the sponge at the site of bleeding.

A flexible, fiberoptic bronchoscope can also be used to deliver fibrin sealant to the tracheobronchial tree using a silastic catheter through the biopsy channel of the bronchoscope [3]. Fibrinogen is initially deposited under direct vision at the desired location via the silastic catheter, followed by the delivery of bovine thrombin. Fibrin sealant can be applied even through an arterial catheterization system at the time of catheter removal to reduce the likelihood of arterial hemorrhage. This system may allow for the early mobilization of patients postcatheterization. It may also allow for safer management of heparinized patients requiring removal of femoral catheters or intra-aortic balloon pumps.

## TCV USES OF FIBRIN SEALANT

A wide variety of clinical uses for fibrin sealant exists in TCV surgery. Fibrin sealant, with success rates varying from 88% to 100% can be used to control the leakage of air, blood, or fluid.

For reduction of air leaks fibrin sealant can be applied to raw lung surfaces [6], as well as pulmonary and bronchial staple lines [7]. In addition, bronchopleural fistulas treated with [3] or without [8,9] the flexible fiberoptic bronchoscope and pneumothoraces treated via the thorascope [10] or chest tube [11] can be managed using fibrin sealant.

An even broader variety of applications exists for control of hemorrhage. Uses include: spray application with or without a carrier sponge for mediastinal bleeding following initial [12] or reoperative cardiac procedures; reinforcement of complex or inaccessible suture lines in congenital or adult cardiac cases [5]; sealing of vascular grafts and anastomoses in aneurysm or dissection repairs [13]; and reinforcement of cardiac patches [14,15] and catheter or cannula insertion sites [5]. It has been used to control bleeding from the bronchial tree [16] and chest wall [5].

Fibrin sealant can also be employed to reduce leakage of other body fluids in TCV. These applications include: reinforcement of esophageal staple lines following anastomoses [5], closure of tracheoesophageal fistulas [17], and control of chylothoraces [18].

## RECENT INNOVATIONS

As use of fibrin sealant increases in this country, innovative uses in thoracic and cardiovascular procedures are to be anticipated. A number of recent authors have attempted to enhance the development and use of autologous [19,21] or even bovine [22] fibrinogen. Methods of reducing sealant fibrinolysis using antifibrinolytic agents when longer-term survival of the adhesive is desirable are also well-known [23]. Application of fibrin sealant as a slow delivery system for antibiotic release is also under active investigation [24].

## COMPLICATIONS

The risks of fibrin-sealant use must be always kept in mind. Beyond the issue of blood-borne disease transmission, other complications have been reported. These include hemodynamic effects [25], anaphylaxis [26], and production of antibodies to human coagulation factors [27,28]. These complications may, however, be related, at least in part, to the use of bovine thrombin required to produce fibrin sealant. Efforts to develop human thrombin sources are in progress in order to reduce some of these dangers. The issue of tissue fibrosis in response to fibrin sealant application has been evaluated and, at least in situations where sealant is used without antifibrinolytics, does not appear to be clinically significant [29].

## CONCLUSION

The use of fibrin sealant as a tissue adhesive in thoracic and cardiovascular surgery is extensive and includes reduction of air, blood and fluid leakage. A number of different application methods and specific indications for use exist. Further efforts to develop new uses, as well as safer and more effective forms of fibrin sealant, are in progress.

## REFERENCES

1. Spotnitz, W. D., Mintz, P. D., Avery, N., Bithell, T. C., Kaul, S., Nolan, S. P. Fibrin glue from stored human plasma: An inexpensive and efficient method for local blood bank preparation. *Am. Surg.*, 53:460–464, 1987.
2. Baker, J. W., Spotnitz, W. D., Nolan, S. P. A technique for spray application of fibrin glue during cardiac operations. *Ann. Thorac. Surg.*, 43:564–565, 1987.
3. Glover, W., Chavis, T. C., Daniel, T. M., Kron, I. L., Spotnitz, W. D. Fibrin glue application via the flexible fiberoptic bronchoscope: Closure of bronchopleural fistulas. *J. Thorac. Cardiovasc. Surg.*, 93:470–472, 1987.
4. Ismail, S., Combs, M. J., Goodman, N. C., Teates, C. D., Abbott, R. D., Nolan, S. P., Teotia, S., Fechner, R. E., Powers, E. R., Spotnitz, W. D. Reduction of femoral arterial bleeding postcatheterization using percutaneous application of fibrin sealant, 1995.
5. Matthew, T. L., Spotnitz, W. D., Kron, I. L., Daniel, T. M. Tribble, C. G., Nolan, S. P. Four years' experience with fibrin sealant in thoracic and cardiovascular surgery. *Ann. Thorac. Surg.*, 50:40–44, 1990.
6. Vincent, J. G., Van De Wal, H. J., Meijer, J. M., Van Herwaarden, C., Lacquet, L. K. Postponing the limits. Multiple and repeated pulmonary metastasectomy by parenchymal sparing electrocautery excision. *Helv. Chir. Acta,* 57:295–300, 1990.
7. Mouritzen, C., Dromer, K., Keinecke, H. O. The effects of fibrin gluing to seal bronchial and alveolar leakages after pulmonary resections and decortications. *Eur. J. Cardiothorac. Surg.*, 7:75–80, 1993.
8. Nicholas, J. M., Dulchavsky, S. A. Successful use of autologous fibrin gel in traumatic bronchopleural fistula: A case report. *J. Trauma,* 32:87–88, 1992.
9. Salmon, C. J., Pon, R. B., Westcott, J. L. Endobronchial vascular occlusion coils for control of a large parenchymal bronchopleural fistula. *Chest,* 98:233–234, 1990.
10. Hauck, H., Bull, P. G., Pridun, N. Complicated pneumothorax: Short- and long-term results of endoscopic fibrin pleurodesis. *World J. Surg.*, 15:146–150, 1991.
11. Yaduda, Y., Mori, A., Kato, H., Fujino, S., Asakura, S. Intrathoracic fibrin glue for postoperative pleuropulmonary fistula. *Ann. Thorac. Surg.*, 51:242–244, 1991.

12. Spotnitz, W. D., Dalton, M. S., Baker, J. W., Nolan, S. P. Reduction of preoperative hemorrhage by anterior mediastinal spray application of fibrin glue during cardiac operations. *Ann. Thorac. Surg.*, 44:529–531, 1987.
13. Dottori, V., Spagnolo, S., Passerone, G., Lijoi, A., Barberis, L., Agostini, M., DeGaetano, G., Paordi, E., Maccario, M., Fumagalli, E. C. Ten years of surgery of aortic dissections and aneurysms: Clinical experience and original conditions. *Minerva Cardioangio.*, 40:431–436, 1992.
14. Zongo, M., La Canna, G., Ceconi, C., Gerrari, M., Latini, L., Lorusso, R., Sandrelli, L., Alfieri, O. Postinfarction left ventricular free wall rupture: Original management and surgical technique. *J. Card. Surg.*, 6:396–399, 1991.
15. Seguin, J. R., Frapier, J. M., Colson, P., Chaptal, P. A. Fibrin sealant for early repair of acquired ventricular septal defect. *J. Thorac. Cardiovasc. Surg.*, 104:748–751, 1992.
16. Bense, L. Intrabronchial selective coagulative treatment of hemoptysis: Report of three cases. *Chest,* 97:990–996, 1990.
17. Antonelli, M., Cicconetti, F., Vivino, G., Gasparetto, A. Closure of a tracheoesophageal fistula by bronchoscopic application of fibrin glue and decontamination of the oral cavity. *Chest,* 100:578–579, 1991.
18. Shirai, T., Amano, J., Takabe, K. Thoracoscopic diagnosis and treatment of chylothorax after pneumonectomy. *Ann. Thorac. Surg.*, 52:306–307, 1991.
19. Kjaergard, H. K., Weis-Fogh, U., Sorensen, H., Thiis, J., Rygg, I. Autologous fibrin glue preparation and clinical use in thoracic surgery. *Eur. J. Cardiothorac. Surg.*, 6:52–54, 1992.
20. Oz, M. C., Jeevanadam, V., Smith, C. R., Williams, M. R., Kaynar, A. M., Frank, R. A., Mosca, R., Reiss, R. F., Rose, E. A. Autologous fibrin glue from intraoperatively collected platelet-rich plasma. *Ann. Thorac. Surg.*, 53:530–531, 1992.
21. Kjaergard, H. K., Weis-Fogh, U. S., Thiis, J. J. Preparation of autologous fibrin glue from pericardial blood. *Ann. Thorac. Surg.*, 55:543–544, 1993.
22. Ismail, S., Glasheen, W. P., Gonias, S. L., Jane, J. A., Spotnitz, W. D. Bovine fibrin sealant: The intraperitoneal life span of a new hemostatic agent. *Surgical Forum* ( In press, 1995).
23. Pipan, C. M., Glasheen, W. P., Matthew, T. L., Gonias, S. L., Hwang, L. J., Jane, J. A., Spotnitz, W. D. Effects of antifibrinolytic agents on the life span of fibrin sealant. *J. Surg. Res.*, 53:402–407, 1992.
24. Kram, H. B., Bansul, M., Timberlake, O., et al. Antibacterial effects of fibrin glue on fibrin glue-antibiotic mixtures. *Trans. Soc. Biomat.*, 12:164, 1989.
25. Kanchuger, M. S., Eide, T. R., Mancke, G. R., Hartman, A., Poppers, P. J. The hemodynamic effects of topical fibrin glue during cardiac operations. *J. Cardiothorac. Anesth.*, 3:745–747, 1989.
26. Milde, L. N. An anaphylactic reaction to fibrin glue. *Anesth. Analg.*, 69:684–686, 1989.
27. Rapaport, I. S., Zivelin, A., Minow, R. A., Huner, C. S., Donnelly, K. Clinical significance of antibodies to bovine and human thrombin and factor V after surgical use of bovine thrombin. *Am. J. Clin. Pathol.*, 97:84–91, 1992.
28. Berruyer, M., Amiral, J., Ffrench, P., Belleville, J., Bastien, O., Clerc, J.,

Kassir, A., Estanove, S., Dechavanne, M. Immunization by bovine thrombin used with fibrin glue during cardiovascular operations: Development of thrombin and factor V inhibitors. *J. Thorac. Cardiovasc. Surg.*, 105:892–897, 1993.

29. Baker, J. W., Spotnitz, W. D., Matthew, T. L., Fechner, R. E., Nolan, S. P. Mediastinal fibrin glue: Hemostatic effect and tissue response in calves. *Ann. Thorac. Surg.*, 47:450–452, 1989.

# INDEX